One Little Miracle

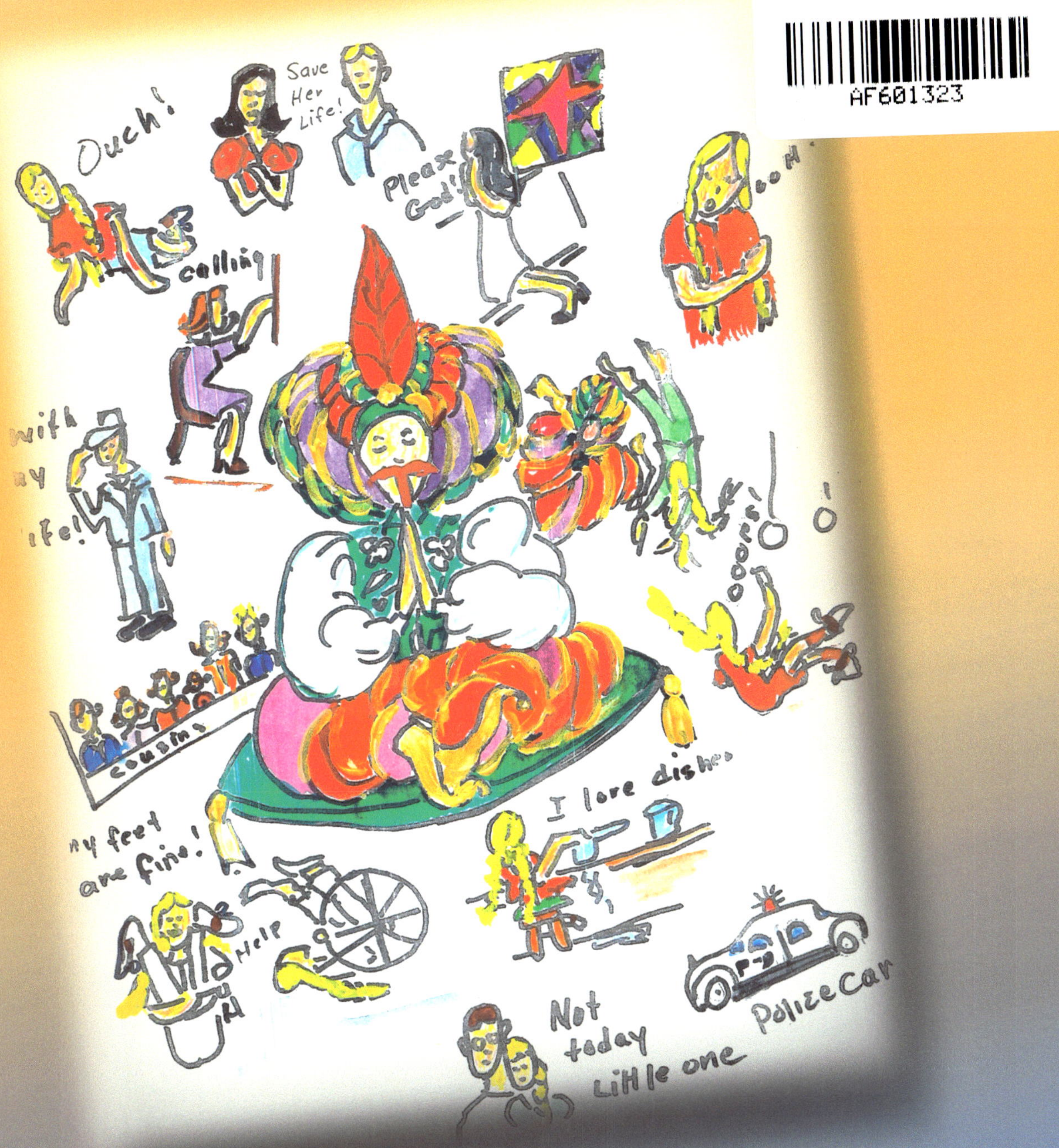

Yvonne Nunes

Library of Congress Control Number: 2010908466
ISBN: Softcover 978-1-4535-1780-2
Hardcover 978-1-4535-1781-9

This book was printed in the United States of America.

To order additional copies of this book, contact:
Xlibris Corporation
1-888-795-4274
www.Xlibris.com
Orders@Xlibris.com

Acknowledgments

Thanks are extended to all my friends in the art club, neighborhood, and monthly dinner group. Norm, my instructor, suggested writing would be easier if I learned to type. Later he said forget the typing. You need Dragon NaturallySpeaking. I'm not a typist, but I certainly have no problem talking. Thank you, Norm. You made my life much easier. I could not have written this book without your help and support. Pat, Dale, and Cherie critiqued the book. You found all the mistakes I couldn't. Claudette, Don, Jerry, and Kenneth—my siblings—and their families have supported me all their lives. Thank you for your honesty and love.

To those of you who have read or listened to part of the manuscript: Pat, the art club group, Norm, Helga and Dale, Monica, Bruce and John, Mary, Janice. Merel and Carol, I loved our day together. Your enthusiasm and encouragement have made writing this book a fascinating visit to my past. I also want to thank the class at Sierra College for the publishing information and your encouragement and support. The Xlibris support people have been very helpful, patient, and supportive. Thank you, all!

Prologue

This is my story. It happened a long time ago when I was seven years old. I am telling and illustrating my story as though I were the age I was when all these things happened. The year was 1943. The world was at war. Most of the countries in Europe and many of the countries in Asia were embroiled in a horrible shooting, fighting, burning war. The war was called World War II.

The United States, where I lived, was on war effort status. Nearly all of the young men were drafted into military service. Some went to Europe. Other young men in the service fought on the islands of the Pacific Ocean and much of Asia.

The war effort made it impossible to buy a car because automakers were building tanks, trucks, jeeps, and vehicles to support our troops who were fighting the war. Gasoline was rationed, so if you had a car, you were limited to the amount of gas you could buy to run your car. Many people did not own their own car. People walked, rode with people who had cars, took a bus, train, or taxi to get where they needed to go.

Food like milk, eggs, and meat were also rationed. Each family had ration stamps for the things they needed. Rationing was done to allow everyone to share what was available. Every person in the family was counted. If you had a large family, you got more ration stamps. If the family was small, it needed fewer ration stamps. That way no one went without food.

Telephones were a luxury. Only about half the homes in the country had telephones. If people did have a telephone in their home, they usually shared a party line. A telephone party line means that many different people use the same line. You could have as many as thirteen families using the same telephone line. If you tried to make a phone call, you hoped that nobody else was on the line. If the line was being used by one of the other thirteen families when you try to call, the proper etiquette would be to hang up and call later. Most people were polite, and if they knew that someone else needed to make a call, they would end their conversation and get off the line. Many times, when two people wanted to use the phone at the same time, they would visit a minute with the other person who shared their line. If you wanted to make a phone call out of town, you called the telephone operator. You would give her the number you want her to call, and she would place your call. If you wanted to call out of the state or a long distance, it could take hours to finally make your call. The reason it took so long was because the operator had to call several operators to find the one who could place your call in that area.

In 1943, most of the people in the United States lived in the country. Some people lived on large farms that supplied food to towns and cities all over the country. Some people lived on small pieces of land where they might have a cow, a garden, and some chickens on the edge of towns. Many homes in the country did not have indoor bathrooms. Outdoor bathrooms were called *outhouses*. They were a lot like porta-potties that are used today in some wilderness areas. Baths were taken in large portable tubs in the back porch or in the kitchen. Some families had washing machines, but nobody had a dryer. Clothes were hung out to dry.

There were very few major highways. Transporting food and materials around the country was done by the railroad. Most people who traveled far would travel by train. Trucks would transport products from farms and factories to the train.

Most of the young men were drafted into military service to fight in the war. But there were some young men who were deferred from the military because the war effort included keeping the trains running to move military personnel from one base to another; keeping the cities and towns supplied with food and clothing for the military and civilians; and producing steel for ships, jeeps, trucks, airplanes, guns, ammunition, and other material used to support and move the armed forces. My father and his two brothers were all railroad men. They did not have to go into the military. They worked sixteen hours a day, every day of the week. My father was a boilermaker for the steam engines on the railroad. In 1943, almost all of the trains were moved by steam engines. The boilermaker was the man on the railroad who had to go into the engine's firebox, tear out all the old bricks while they were still hot, and replace them with new firebricks so they could build up the heat to make the steam move the engines. My uncle Alfred was a machinist on the railroad. It was his job to see that all the moving parts were in good repair to move the engine. Uncle Adrian was an engineer on the railroad. He was the man who drove the train. Some farmers were deferred from military service because the world needed food, and they produced it. There were other strategic jobs that needed well-trained civilians to run this country.

In 1943, there were no televisions. We did enjoy our programs, but they were delivered to us through a radio. The other important entertainment that we enjoyed was the movies. Everybody went to the movies. You could go to a movie for one dime, and it cost a nickel for a bag of popcorn. All the kids in Portola would go to the Saturday afternoon matinee.

These are just a few ways life was different between 1943 and 2010. There weren't very many rich people in 1943. I don't think I knew any rich people. But I didn't know any poor people either. Everybody that I knew did the same things that my family did. The one exception, which made us very lucky, was that my father and his two brothers didn't have to go to war. They were deferred because they were needed by the railroad. They worked long hours and very hard, but they were not far away from home in dangerous places. Some of my uncles worked on farms. I did have two uncles in the military. Uncle Albert was in the army. Uncle Joe was in the navy. Uncle Albert served in the Pacific. He would go off the ship with the first wave of soldiers moving on to an island. When they got to the island, the soldiers would try to secure the area by shooting guns to scare the enemy away from the area where they were landing. My uncle Albert's job was to get tractors and trucks dropped by airplanes or off the ship to make a landing field for airplanes to drop supplies to the soldiers fighting the war and take the injured to get medical help. My uncle Joe served on navy bases in the United States. Both of my uncles survived the war.

Strangely, my story was part of the war effort. During terrible fighting all over the world, I had a simple fall. I broke my arm. The bones came out of the skin and picked up one of the most deadly bacteria known to the world at that time. It is called gas gangrene. Gas gangrene was a very common bacteria in the South Pacific where many soldiers, sailors, and marines were fighting. More military personnel were being killed by infection than by bullets at this time. Finding a substance that could kill bacteria could save more lives than what were lost in World War II. I was the first person to survive who had gas gangrene that penetrated the entire body. The only reason I survived is because I was able to get the new drug called penicillin; it killed the gas gangrene. I lived to tell this story.

The players in this drama include:

Dr. Alexander Fleming: A bacteriologist who discovered a substance purely by accident that could, under very controlled conditions in the laboratory, kill bacteria. He was the first person to discover that anything could kill bacteria.

Yvonne Tibbedeaux: A seven-year-old girl who fell and broke her arm in Portola, California. She sustained a compound fracture of her lower left arm. The wound became infected with a deadly bacterial infection—gas gangrene.

Dr. McKnight: A general practitioner working at the Western Pacific Railroad hospital in Portola, California. He cared for Yvonne's injured arm. He set the broken bones. He discovered the cast was too tight and cut it so there could be better air circulation around the wound. The infection became obvious. It was gas gangrene. The cast was removed, and every medical intervention known at that time was performed, including amputation to the shoulder. Still the infection raged through her body. The bacteria was rare; a gas gangrene diagnosis had not been made in the area in over twenty years. Dr. McKnight knew that a search for gas gangrene infection was a high priority for the military. The *JAMA* had sent out a call to doctors for any gas gangrene infection that could be used to test a new drug called penicillin. The specifications were that the patient must have had every known intervention to heal the infection, but the infected person was still losing ground. In other words, in order to get penicillin, the patient had to be dying of a gangrene infection.

Dr. Kiefer: In Boston, was the person to contact in order to be considered part of a penicillin test case to determine if penicillin could destroy the gas gangrene bacteria. There was no medicine known to man that could kill bacteria. There was so little penicillin; the test case had to be a serious gas gangrene infection, which could not be cured any other way.

A general in Washington DC: The last person that had to be contacted in order to have the penicillin released for the test case. He had the power to send penicillin to the person anywhere in the United States who had the infection that could test penicillin. The military was in charge of making this decision because the greatest need for this test case was to save the lives of the men on the battlefield all over the world.

A military Secret Service person: It was his responsibility to contact and inform a railroad conductor that he was needed to transport this valuable cargo.

The conductor: Swore that he would protect the package with his life. He was deputized and armed and received the package. The conductor was told by the Secret Service person that he was carrying the most valuable cargo in the United States.

Genie: The dream friend/playmate who guided Yvonne on magical adventures into a world where everything is possible and *no* is not a word. Yvonne loved Genie.

Mae Tibbedeaux: My aunt who stayed on the phone as the telephone operator for nearly twenty-four hours in order to contact the people who could release penicillin to Dr. McKnight to see if penicillin could kill the gas gangrene.

Family and friends: Cared for me while I was sick, supported my parents in every way they could. They will never be forgotten by my family and me.

Chapter 1

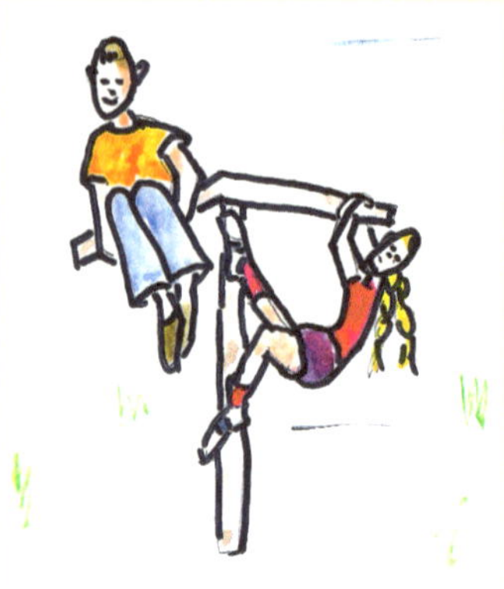

It had been a sweltering hot day in August 1943. My sister, Tyke, and I had played quiet games in the house because it was too hot outside. The day seemed very long. I was bored. I didn't like being in the house playing games. Finally, after dinner, our mother let us go outside.

The evening was cooler, and we went outside to play. Some kids were climbing on the clothesline pole. The clothesline was located toward the back of the apartment house. Tyke didn't like to climb, so she went back in the house. My friend and I climbed up the pole and sat at the top talking about going to school, teachers, things we liked to do, and whatever kids talk about. We were both seven years old.

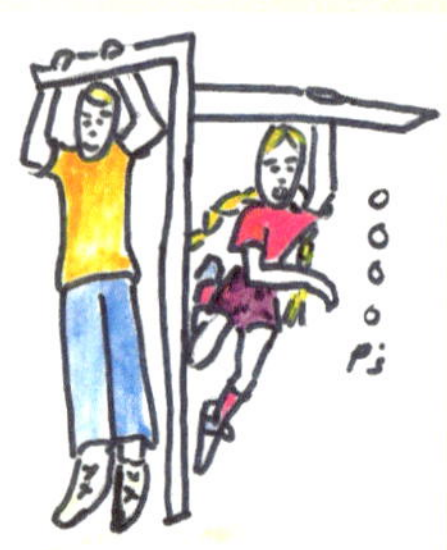

Just before dark, Tyke called me. It was time to come in. I decided to drop down from the bar I was sitting on, which held the clothesline. When I did, my right hand slipped. My left arm twisted while holding on to the bar. The bones in my left arm snapped. I will never forget the snapping sound. I fell to the ground. I remember the pain was excruciating, and I was screaming my head off. I was screaming partly because it hurt and partly because I could see the bones coming out of my arm. This was a *real* broken arm. I was very frightened and in a lot of pain. I knew arms had bones, but I had never seen mine before. My sister had gone back into the house after she called me. She didn't know I was hurt.

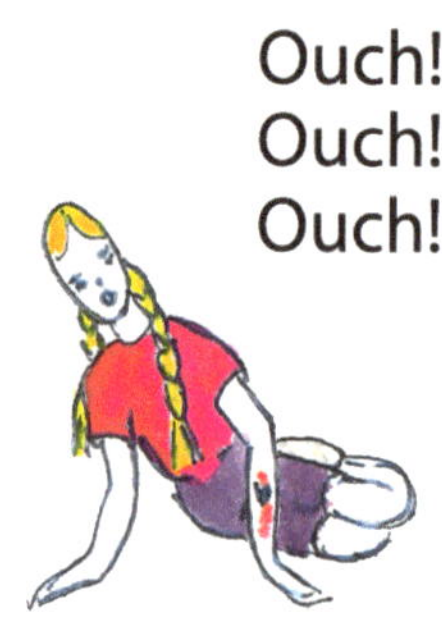

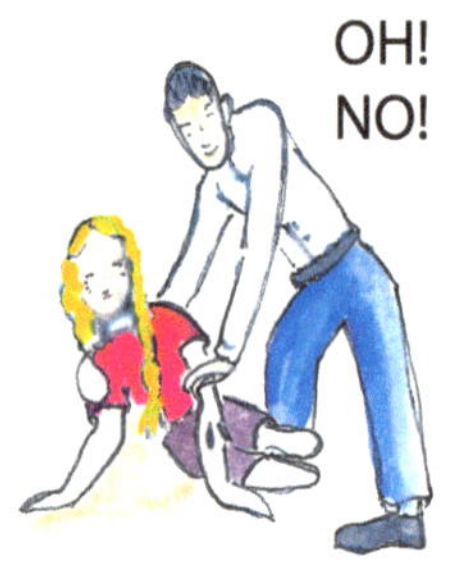

A man walking down the alley behind the apartment heard me and came over to see why I was crying. The man didn't know that my arm was injured. He just knew I was hurt and came to help. He reached down to pick me up and grabbed my broken arm. I screamed. He saw my arm was broken. He said, "I am so sorry." Then he carefully picked me up and carried me home. My mother heard me yelling and came out to see what was going on. When she saw my arm, she covered her mouth with her hands and said, "Oh my god!"

We didn't have a car. We didn't have a telephone either. None of our neighbors had cars or telephones. The telephone office was just down the street. My mother asked a neighbor to go to the telephone office and call my aunt who had a car and a telephone and ask if she could take me to the hospital.

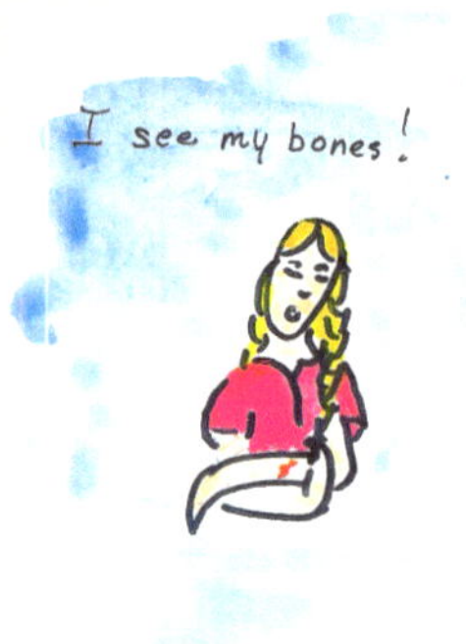

By this time, I had stopped crying. I wanted to look at my arm. Bones coming out of your arm look a little bit like teeth. They are the same color as teeth, and they hurt like teeth, but they're not the same shape. They looked very much like broken teeth. It is very interesting to look at bones. There was not much blood, so I thought I would be okay. My arm looked unreal. It was swollen and bruised. There was dried black blood and a little red blood around the bones. I couldn't tell if I had broken two bones or one broken bone with two ends sticking out. I was feeling very tired and sore. I wanted the doctor to fix my arm to make it stop hurting. I wanted to lie down and go to sleep.

Finally, my aunt Mae got to our house. Mae jumped out of the car, looked at my arm, and asked me how in the world I had done that to myself. I just looked at her. Mae said, "Stupid question, right?" Then she said, "Let's get you into the car and to the hospital."

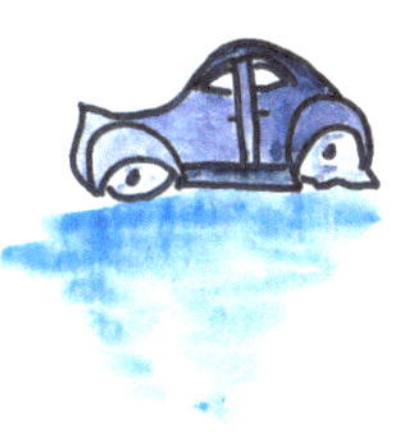

The man who brought me home after my fall picked me up and put me in the car. My mother, my aunt, my sister, and I were in the car when we discovered that the car had a flat tire. My mother said, "I can't believe this is happening." Everybody got out of the car. My aunt ran to the telephone office and called the Western Pacific Hospital. The doctor was not in that evening, but there was a technician who had a car, and he would come and take me to the hospital.

Dr. Loewenberg roared up the road to our house, jumped out of his car, and asked to see the patient. When he looked at my arm, he put his hand under the wound. He was very careful and gentle. He asked me if it hurt. I said, "Yes, it hurts a lot." He said, "Let's get you to the hospital."

He explained to my mother that he was a Jewish refugee from Germany where he had been a doctor. He worked as a technician in California because he was not yet certified as a doctor in this country.

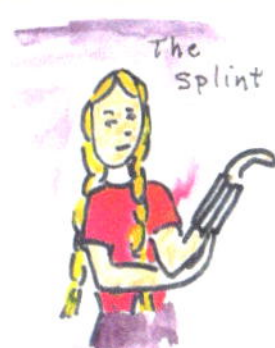

Dr. Loewenberg took me to the hospital where he set my arm in splints. He said the break was too serious for splints, but he was not yet licensed to operate. He was very concerned about the bones coming through the skin. He washed my arm from fingers to shoulder with a disinfectant. He gave me pain medicine and drove us home. He told Mom to bring me back to the hospital first thing in the morning.

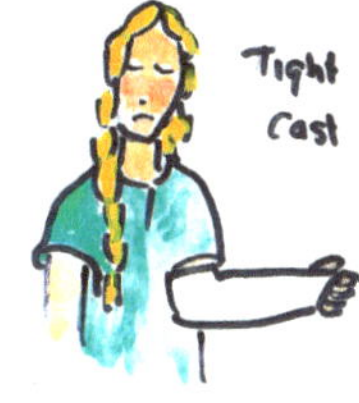

Needless to say, no one in our house slept well that night. I was very uncomfortable, and my parents were very worried. The next morning, they took me to the hospital, and Dr. McKnight set my arm. After the surgery, he told my parents he was very concerned that he had to set the cast tightly to hold the bones in place. He was worried about a lack of blood flow and air circulation around the wound. He decided to have me stay in the hospital overnight for observation.

The next morning, my parents came to visit me at the hospital. They met with the doctor while he was checking my arm. He was concerned about the tight cast. He explained to my parents that he was going to cut the cast to allow better circulation. He warned my parents that my arm might hurt more because of the circulation and to be aware of any changes in my feeling or attitude. The rest of that day and most of the night, I was very uncomfortable. It wasn't until about midnight when I finally fell asleep. When I slept, everyone else went to sleep.

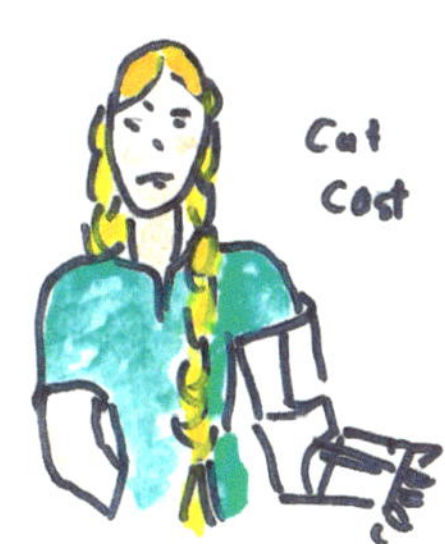

The morning of the third day after my accident, my arm looked worse than it had any time previously. I could only see my fingers because of the cast, but what I could see was frightening. My fingers were reddish, purplish, blotchy blue and as big as sausages. I said, "Look, Mom, look at my hand. My fingers look weird, but they don't hurt anymore." Mom did not smile. She looked carefully at my hand. She was worried that my fingers were too big, the wrong color, and they didn't hurt anymore. That was the really scary thing; my arm didn't hurt anymore. Once again, I was rushed to the doctor at the hospital.

When the doctor saw me that morning, he expressed great concern about my arm. He explained to my mother that the circulation was not good, and he was going to have to do surgery to try to stop the infection. When he picked me up to leave the room, my mother asked him if it was gangrene. He looked at her and said, "How did you know?" My mother explained to him that she had read something in *Reader's Digest* about gas gangrene.

This was not good!

Chapter 2

Gas gangrene was a major killer of American soldiers stationed in the South Pacific during World War II. There was no cure for this infection, and it was very common to get gas gangrene from a scratch or splinter and certainly after any kind of wound caused during combat.

Dr. Fleming, a Scottish bacteriologist, discovered a substance that, under very special conditions in the laboratory, could kill bacterial infections like gas gangrene. This substance was the first evidence that bacteria could be killed and might be used to save lives. The problem with the substance they were testing was it could not be made in large batches, and when they tried, the antibacterial substance would die in the test tubes. There was however a small amount being used to test the effects on infections, especially infection that was common to soldiers at war. This substance was called penicillin. From the *Journal of the American Medical Association*, a magazine for doctors about important trends and medical practices as well as the latest medications being used and studied, Dr. McKnight learned about penicillin and the fact that there was an urgent search in the United States to find a patient with a gas gangrene infection.

When Dr. McKnight discovered that the infection was gas gangrene, he told my parents that he had to perform surgery on my arm. In 1943, the only method of fighting gas gangrene was to make incisions around the infected area from the skin to the bone with the hope that the infection could be killed with better circulation of air. In my case, seven incisions from my elbow to my wrist as well as from skin to bone were needed. There was no medication known that could stop gas gangrene. Dr. McKnight explained the seriousness of the infection to my parents and told them the prescribed procedure for attacking the infection. He then personally carried me into the operating room.

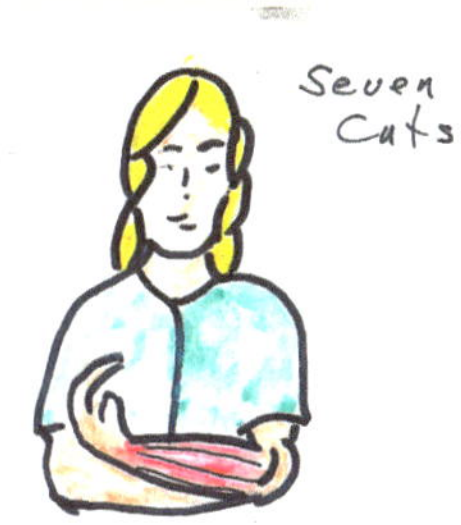

After the surgery, the doctor told my parents the situation was most grave. The infection had reached the bone and was moving up my arm rapidly. There was nothing he could do but hope, pray, and wait. He told my parents to go home because "Yvonne needs rest and so do you."

The next morning, the fourth day after my accident, my parents came to the hospital to see me. The doctor was waiting for them. He told them the infection was moving rapidly and invading my entire body. There was very little hope that I would survive. The doctor told my parents the only chance of survival was for him to amputate my arm just below the shoulder. The hope was that by cutting the infection off my arm, if the gangrene was not too invasive, I might live. For that reason, the sooner the source of the infection was removed, the better my chances of survival would be.

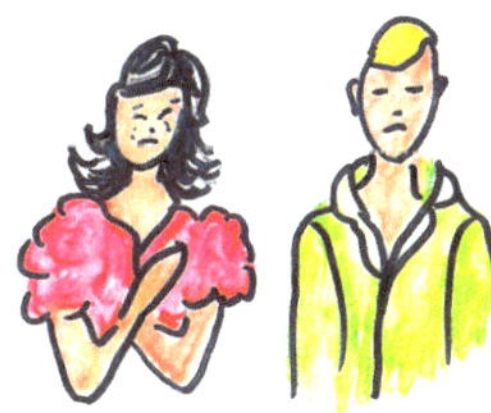

My parents were stunned! They could not imagine this happening to their child. My mother said no! She would rather see her child dead than with one arm. My father looked at the doctor and asked, "Is there no other hope?" The doctor replied, "There is nothing anyone can do for her now except to remove the source of the infection and pray." My father approached my mother; she would not let him touch her. My father asked, "How do we do this?" The doctor answered, "There are papers that must be signed." My mother said she would not sign. My father added, "We have no choice. We'll do whatever we have to do to save Yvonne's life." The decision was made; the forms were signed by both my parents, and the surgery was done.

One of the serious complications of amputations is the danger of hemorrhage. It is important to have a supply of blood that matches the type of the amputee. Although type O is the universal donor for transfusion, in a case of amputation where serious infection is involved and a great loss of blood has taken place, it is dangerous to use anything but the same blood type. My father was type AB+. My mother was type O+. I was type B+. My parents were not a good match. Dr. McKnight sent out a request to everyone in the little town of Portola asking if there was a B+ donor in case blood was needed. No donor was found. Plasma is a solution used to keep veins open to maintain circulation and blood pressure instead of whole blood. Open veins are the passageway to deliver required medicines into the patient's body when the patient can't take them by mouth. Later I was told that my veins had collapsed. When an arm is amputated, arteries and veins are severed causing a lot of blood to drain out of the body. When there is not enough blood flowing through the vein, it goes flat like a tire without air. A *cutdown* is a procedure to find a vein by cutting through the skin and literally holding the vein over the finger of a nurse to get a needle into the vein without going through the vein. When they collapse, it means that there is not enough blood in the veins to circulate through the body to keep blood pressure normal and the heart beating. My veins were held open with plasma because my blood type was rare, and there was no one who could donate blood for me.

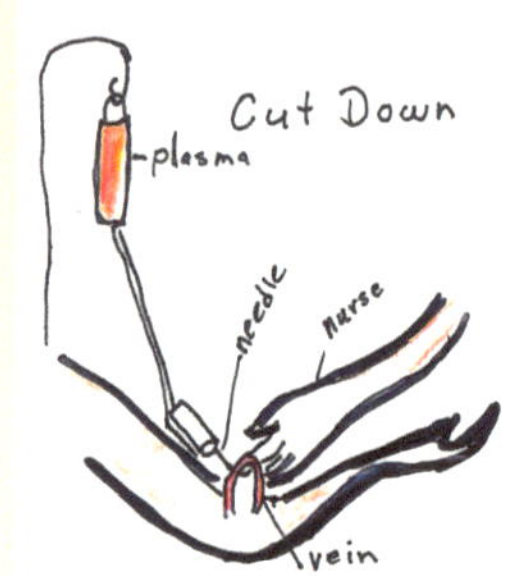

Sometime after the surgery, the first thing I remembered was being wheeled into a room. It was dark because all the shades were drawn, and it was very hot and quiet. The doctor and the nurse were in my room. The doctor was talking to the nurse. He was giving her instructions about how to care for me. This was very interesting to me. He told her to watch me very closely because I might hemorrhage. I didn't know what *hemorrhage* meant, but I knew it was serious by the way he was talking to her. He told her not to leave me for a minute. Don't let her roll over, sit up, or move around. He told the nurse she will probably be too weak to move very much and would probably sleep for a while. Then he left the room. The nurse walked around the room, tucked in my sheet, and bent over to look to see that I was sleeping. I pretended to be asleep. She poured some water in a glass, and then she left the room.

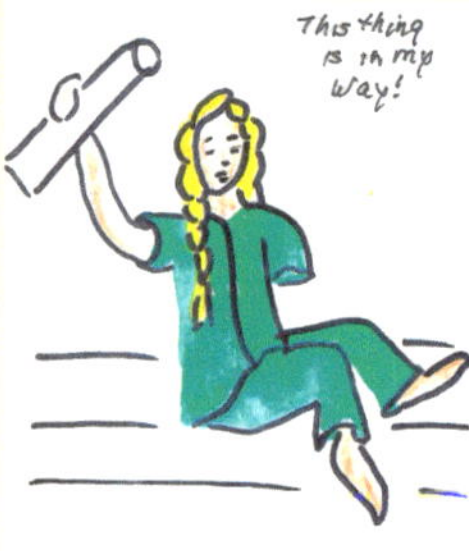

After she left the room, I moved around to see what my arm looked like. My arm was in a big cast. It was too heavy to move. It was hot, and I didn't feel good. It was time to go home. Turning over was impossible because the cast was in my way. Sitting up, in order to see the cast better, I threw it across the room. I was totally unaware that there was no arm in that cast. Sliding slowly out of the bed, first one foot and then both of my feet were on the floor. Dizziness overtook me with a wave of nausea, causing my stomach to turn. I waited to get past the weakness; my head was throbbing. I felt like I was going to be sick. I was trying to hang on to the side of the bed, waiting to feel stronger. After a while, it was time to go. I lifted my head; my head and stomach felt a little better. I walked to the door, went out the door and down the hall toward the front of the hospital. That part of the hall was all glass on one side and very bright. The bright light hurt my eyes. I couldn't see anything. I felt awful. I couldn't wait to get home.

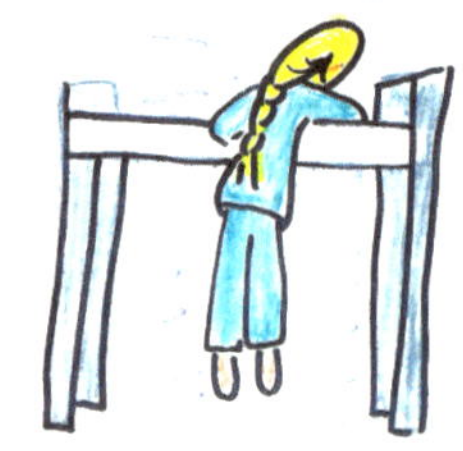

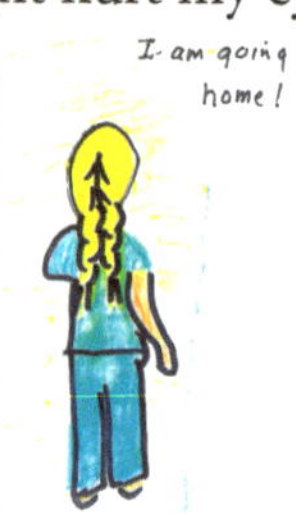

All of a sudden, out of the brightness came Dr. McKnight. He stopped in front of me and said, "What are you doing out of bed?" "I am going home." He picked me up and said, "Not today, little one."

And that was that.

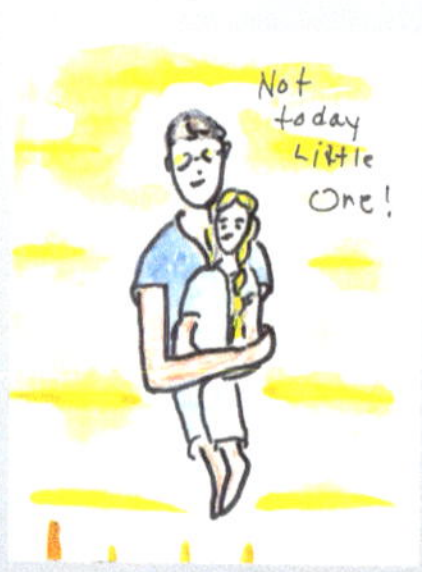

Chapter 3

Dr. McKnight took me back to my room. He called the nurse and asked her why she had left me. She told him that I was asleep, and she just left the room for a minute to get something. Dr. McKnight told her not to leave me until he returned. He went to the secretary of the hospital and asked her to call every church and every woman's club in town for volunteers to sit with me in the hospital. She was to inform the volunteers a little girl was badly hurt and could not be left alone. Volunteers would be needed twenty-four hours a day because Yvonne's mother was eight months pregnant and needed to avoid stress. Before the secretary left the hospital that day, she had volunteers lined up for a week.

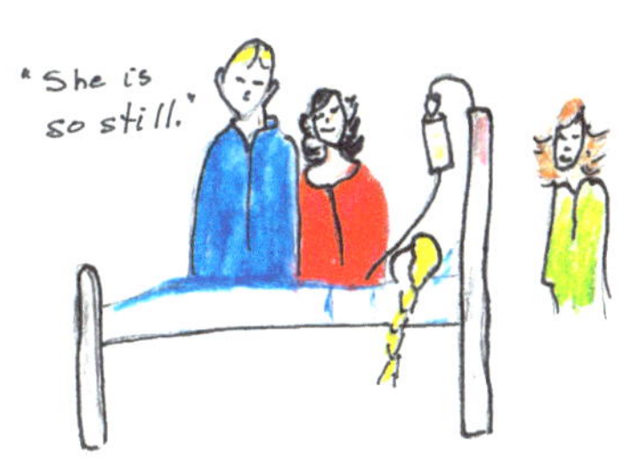

My parents came in to see me the evening after my surgery. A volunteer was sitting with me. She told my mother and father that she would be coming in a few hours every day for the rest of the week. She explained to my mother that the doctor had asked for help to care for Yvonne day and night. Most of the women in town said they were happy to be able to help. My mother was eight months pregnant and very worried about me. She wanted to be at the hospital, but the doctor had told her to stay home. My father was worried about my mother and me. My parents thanked her for her help. Their help was much appreciated.

Dr. McKnight came and talked to my parents that evening. He told them that I was very sick, my fever was high, the infection was raging in my body, and he was going to spend the night at the hospital with me.

During that night, I got sicker. Dr. McKnight had heard of and was interested in a new antibiotic medicine called penicillin. There was very little of this drug available. What he had read in the medical journal was that there was a great need to find a gas gangrene test case for this drug. Gas gangrene was one of the infections that was deadlier than the bullets and bombs being used in the war. American servicemen were dying from gas gangrene infections. Finding a test case was difficult because this infection is rare in the United States.

By early morning of the fourth day after my accident, Dr. McKnight knew there was no way I would survive without a very unusual and immediate intervention. He got the phone number of Dr. Kiefer in Boston. He had found out that Dr. Kiefer was the only person who could release penicillin for patient use. We would get the medication only if it benefited the war effort and the patient had no other possibility of surviving.

Dr. McKnight drove to the telephone office at six o'clock in the morning. He went into the office and asked the telephone operator if she could make a call to Boston, Massachusetts. In 1943, to get a phone call from Portola to Sacramento could take half a day. A phone call from Portola, California to Boston, Massachusetts could take all day and all night. The telephone operator just happened to be my aunt Mae—the aunt who brought the car to take me to the hospital and then had a flat tire. She was just going off duty, but she told the doctor she would stay on the phone until she got Dr. Kiefer or whoever she needed to contact to get the penicillin to Portola.

It took all day, and my aunt finally got Dr. Kiefer in Boston. She told him that Dr. McKnight had requested that she make this call for a little girl who had gangrene in her left arm; the arm had been amputated, but the infection was still raging, and there was no hope of saving this child unless penicillin could kill the infection. Dr. Kiefer told her that he would release all the penicillin they had in the world for a gas gangrene infection. The only problem was that his release had to be approved by a general at the Pentagon in Washington DC. He gave my aunt the name and phone number of the general in Washington DC. My aunt stayed on the phone until two o'clock the next morning to reach him. The general said, "She can have all we've got. The world supply of penicillin has been sent by military aircraft to San Francisco." He asked her how to get it to Portola. My aunt looked at her watch and said, "There is a train leaving San Francisco in twenty minutes." The general said, "It will be on that train. Have a police car with armed police meet the train. Penicillin is the most precious commodity in the world today. And every bit of usable penicillin we have in this country will be in Portola tonight."

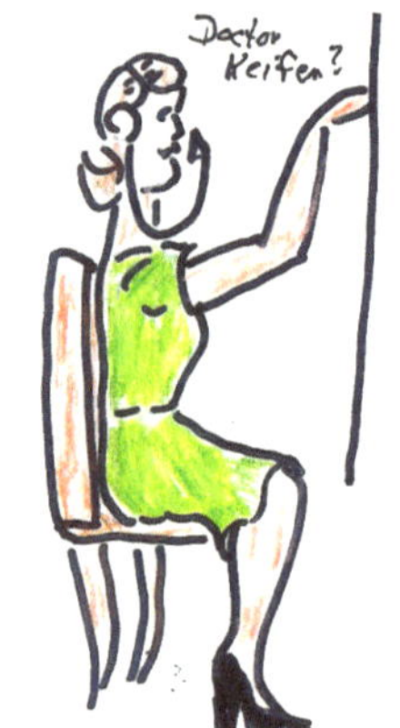

The Western Pacific Railroad was contacted by the military and told that a railroad conductor would be deputized to become a military courier of a top secret package. This railroad conductor would be armed, and the package would be fastened to his body. The conductor, when he was approached by a military officer, said he would proudly protect this package with his life. He was informed that he would be met at the train station in Portola by a police car with armed protection, and he would be transported by police car to the hospital. The conductor was informed that he was carrying the most valuable cargo in the world.

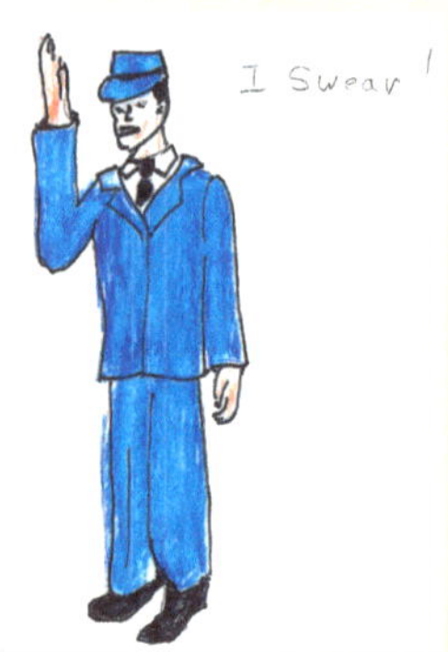

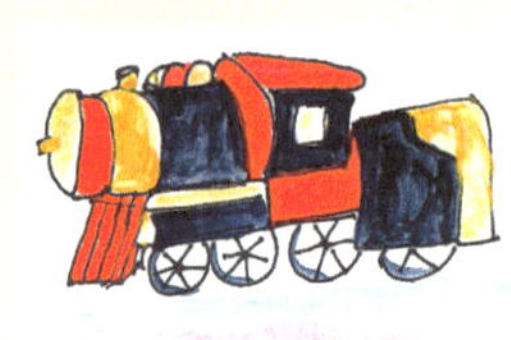
Train

The penicillin arrived with great fanfare. The train station was about half a block from the hospital, but the sirens were blaring, and all the lights were blinking brightly as the only police car in Portola drove its precious cargo with the armed Western Pacific Railroad conductor and police guard to the hospital.

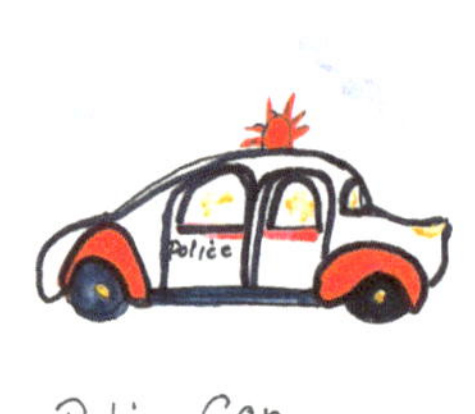

Police Car

In the meantime, my entire body was affected by the infection. My vital signs were weaker; I was comatose and had a dangerously high fever.

The penicillin that arrived that night was not the penicillin that is used today. It was coarse and took a very large hypodermic needle to force it into the body. It looked a little like chicken fat—yellow, viscous, and grainy. Penicillin was introduced in to my body through a drip into a vein in my right arm. When the veins opened enough, hypodermic needles were used to give me a shot every hour, first in one hip and then the other. Dr. McKnight's greatest concern was that the penicillin might be too late. We truly needed a miracle.

All we can do was hope and pray.

Chapter 4

The penicillin had arrived. I was very sick but still alive. They had begun the IV drip in my arm using plasma to open my veins. The first hypodermic injection of penicillin into my hip had also begun. There were volunteers to sit with me twenty-four hours a day. Every church and every woman's club was praying for me.

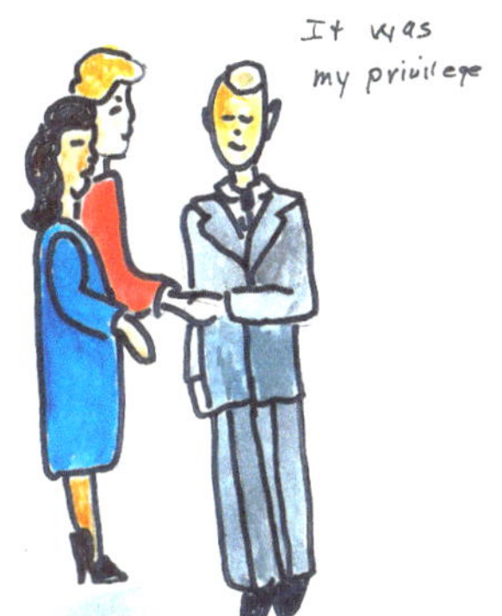

The conductor from the train met with my parents and Dr. McKnight. He said being deputized and armed by the military to deliver penicillin to a tiny mountain town—to save the life of a little girl—was the most important thing he had ever done or probably ever would do in his life.

Everyone was guardedly hopeful that the penicillin would work and I would survive.

The day after the penicillin arrived, I was still comatose; my vital signs were very low, and hope was beginning to wane. My mother was exhausted and feeling very unwell. Dr. McKnight told my mother not to come back to the hospital. He explained to her that it was very important that she take care of herself and her unborn child.

My mother was very upset; she knew why the doctor didn't want her to be there. She didn't want to stay away. My mother's mother and my father's mother both my grandmothers, came to Portola to support my mother and father, take care of my little sister, and do anything they could to help.

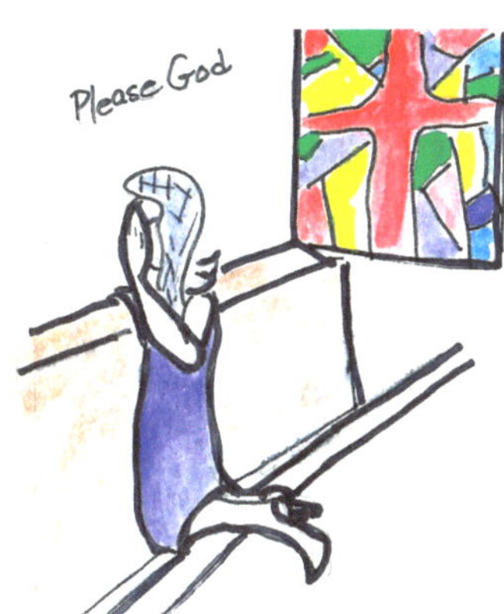

My family suffered emotional swings from great hope to terrible despair. A low time for my mother came when the doctor asked her to stay away from the hospital. The stress was causing a health risk for her and the baby. She was in her eighth month, and she was losing weight. That day, she left the hospital and walked to the church. She went into the church and knelt next to the altar. She cried. She asked God how he could take another child from her. She had lost a little girl just two years before. My little sister, Donna, had died on Valentine's Day. Donna had been one year old. "Please, God, would it be possible to grant us one little miracle to save Yvonne?"

One of the things my grandmothers did was stay with me at the hospital. They both took turns relieving the other volunteers. It was very quiet in my room; nothing much was happening because I was in a coma.

My grandma Nicholes, my father's mother, told me a story that happened while she was with me. She said it was afternoon. The room was dark. The shades were drawn. It was very warm and still. She was sitting by my bed in a rocking chair, and she was dozing. The nurse came into the room with a mirror. She put the mirror near my mouth to see if I was breathing. My grandmother asked her if I was okay. The nurse said, "Yes, she is very quiet, but she is still with us." After the nurse left the room, my grandmother said she watched me, just sat and watched me. She said I was so still, so small and so unmoving. It was unlike the real me

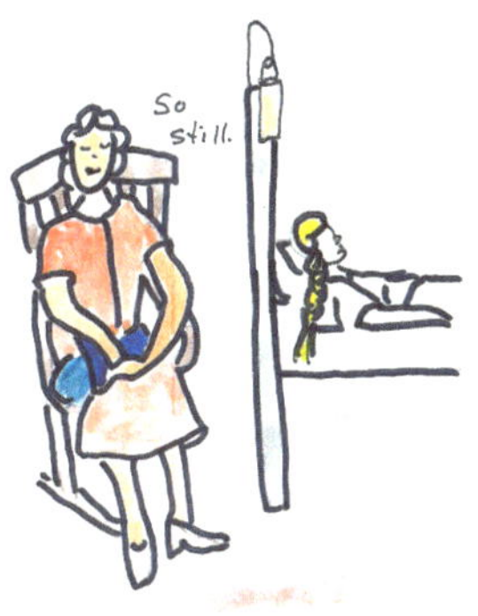

who was never still and never unmoving. She began to doze again. Then something startled her awake. She looked at me. I looked the same. But something was different; my foot was moving. She stood up, came closer to the bed, and looked at my face. I was absolutely still; my face was very pale, but she saw a small pink circle on my cheek, and the circle was growing. She ran to the door and yelled down the hall for the nurse to come immediately. When the nurse got there, my grandmother said, "Look, what is happening?" The nurse started to cry. "Maybe we have our miracle." She ran down the hall to find the doctor.

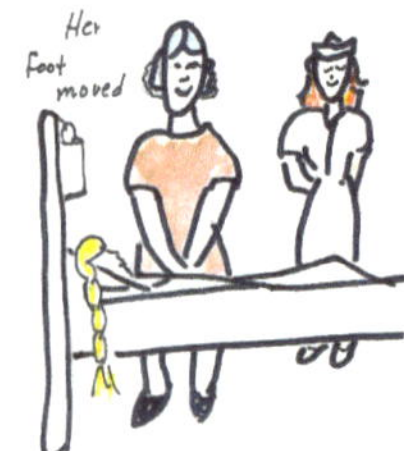

Dr. McKnight and the nurse checked all my vital signs. He told my grandmother that this could possibly be a good sign. My vitals hadn't changed. I was not better yet. He said we probably shouldn't tell my mother in case this episode did not mean that I was getting well. But my grandmother told me later that she knew that the small pink circle was a very good sign that I was getting better.

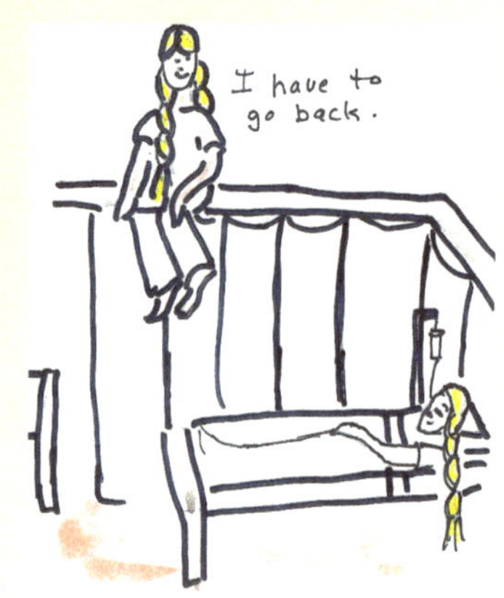

It was about this time. I don't know the sequence or how many days had come or gone, but I remember being alone someplace different from my room. It was a smaller area, barely large enough for my bed, and there were screens all around it with curtains. I was awake, and I was very sick. I felt terrible. My head ached. Everything hurt. I felt awful. There were nurses on the other side of the screen; I could not see them but I could hear them. They were talking about someone. They were saying "her mother can't come to visit her" because they don't want her mother to be there when she dies. They were talking about me! I was furious. How could they say someone was going to die? Who are they? I was sitting on top of the screen and saw three nurses walk out of the room. Suddenly, the realization that sitting on top of the screen was impossible even for me. "How did I get here? That's me in bed. How can a person be in the bed and be sitting on the screen at the same time?" I also began to realize that I didn't hurt or feel sick anymore. I felt good. I wasn't sick. What was happening to me? I liked being higher. I could see a lot more up here. I didn't have to look up at everybody. I could sit up here and look down at me in the bed and at nurses coming in and out of my room. I knew that staying on top of the screen was a very special event. The only option for me was to go back to bed. I didn't want to go back. But if I didn't go back to bed, the nurses would be right, and then maybe I would die. Dying was out of the question. I didn't want to die or be sick anymore. I thought about it for a long time. Maybe climbing down from the top of the screen wouldn't be too hard. It was not very far from the bed. The door was very close to my bed, just a short walk and out the door. What if the nurses were waiting outside the door? They would bring me back to bed. My head ached. Climbing down from the top of the screen seemed impossible. I had to go back to bed, and I was very sick again.

Sometime later (I don't know how many days), I came out of coma—still very sick, unsure of the final outcome—but I was better than I had been, and there was real hope that there would be a complete recovery. Maybe penicillin was a miracle.

Mom could visit me again!

Chapter 5

During the next few days, after the episode with the pink circle on my cheek, I continued to stay about the same. The infection was still present, but it didn't seem to be spreading or getting any worse. It also didn't seem to be going away or getting any better. It was during this time that I remember some very strange and wonderful things happening to me. One of the amazing things I saw and enjoyed was my genie. He was a little man, no bigger than I, with a goatee, mustache, and whiskers. He was dressed in an enormous turban. The turban was made of brilliant, shiny silks, satins, and velvets. It had beautiful colors of magenta, aquamarine, red, and gold. He also had on a glistening white shirt and a vest of aquamarine trimmed with magenta flowers and gold leaves. On both his hands, all of his fingers had rings, beautiful rings of gold with bright colored stones that sparkled. He had striped bloomers of magenta-and-red silk. He sat with his legs crossed on an enormous green silk cushion with gold tassels on all four corners. His feet wore spectacular golden slippers with toes curled over with little gold bells on the tips of his curly-toed shoes. He was my best friend and my greatest joy. He would take me on trips and tell me stories. He made me laugh when we would make fun of all the nurses and doctors and people who came to my room. We laughed uproariously. We rolled and tumbled, giggled and shouted. I loved him. Genie couldn't stay with me all the time. Sometimes he had to leave, but he told me if I really needed him, all I had to do was tell the nurse to bring me a spoonful of water, and then he would come back to play with me. All of my nurses knew about Genie. They couldn't see him, and they couldn't hear him. I told them about him, and they always smiled and told me how lucky I was to have a friend. Whenever I asked the nurse to bring me a spoonful of water, she would do it, and Genie would come. The nurses told me while I was having all this fun with Genie, all they could see was me lying very still as though I were asleep.

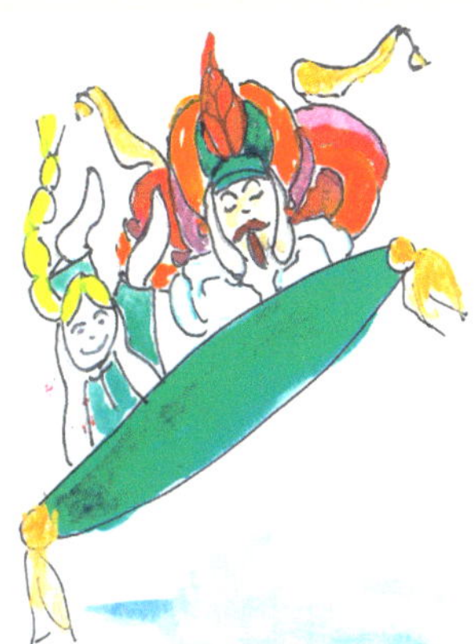

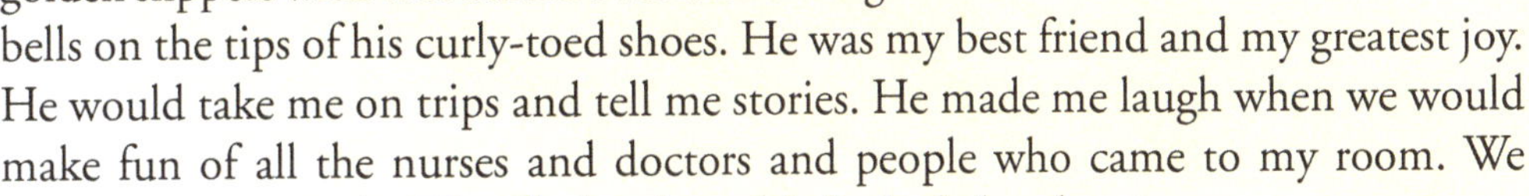

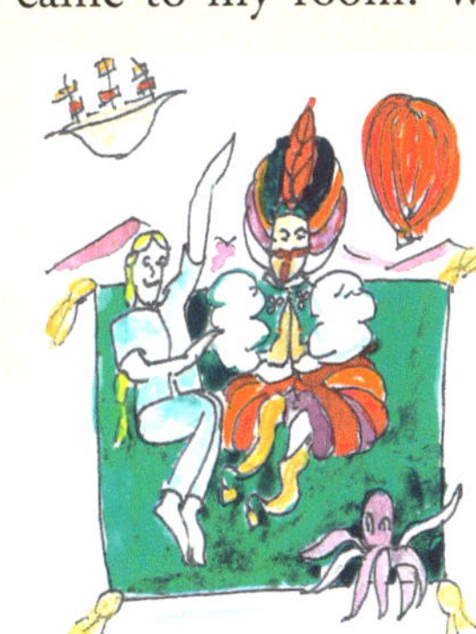

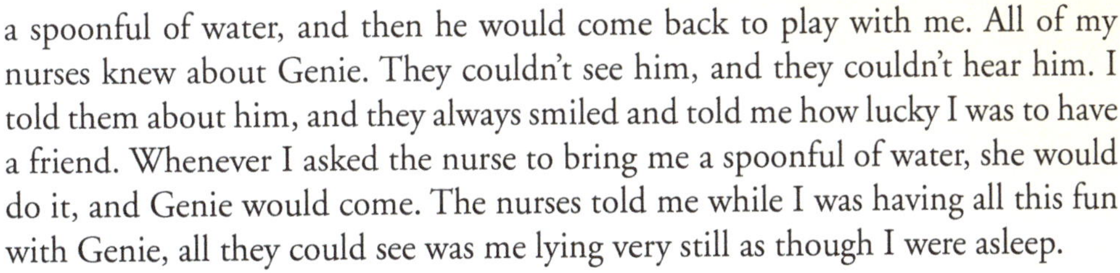

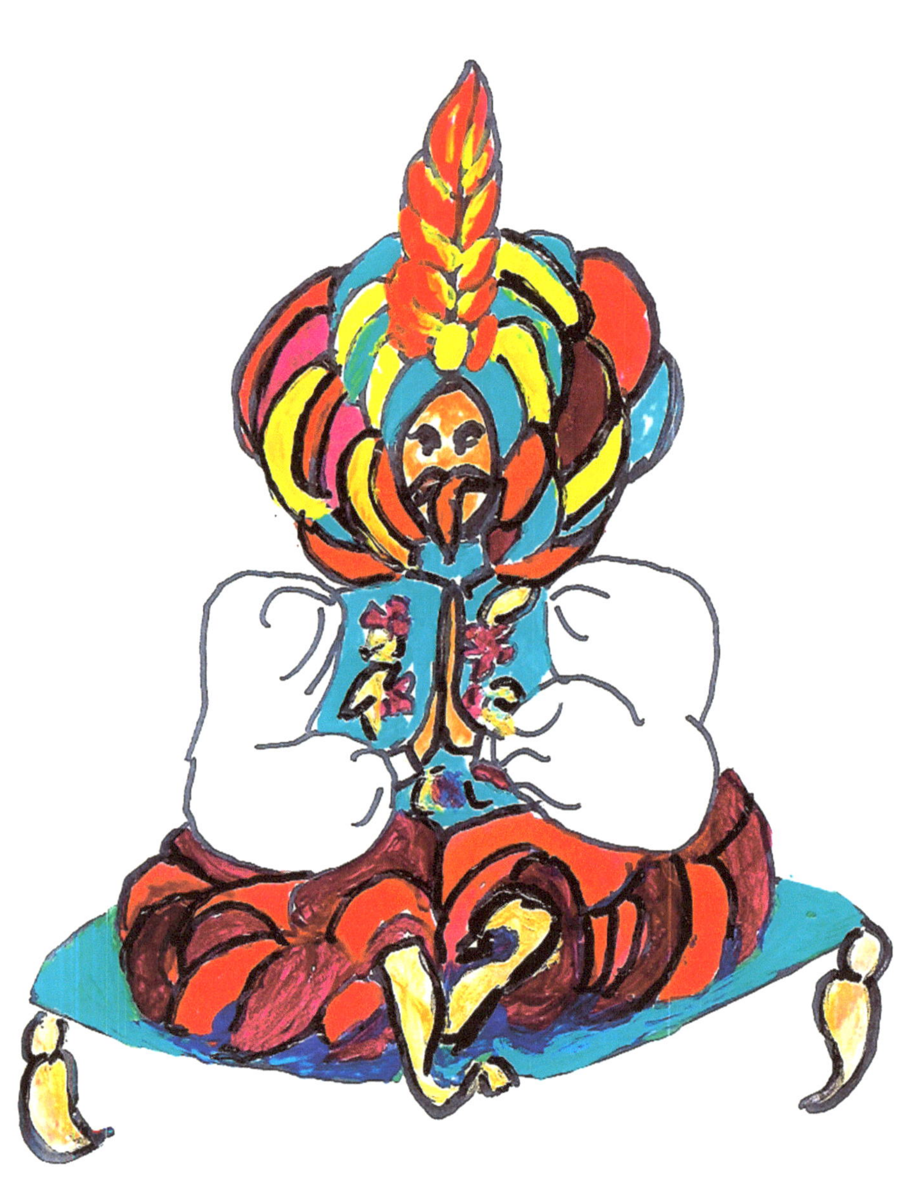

Change is coming!

Chapter 5A

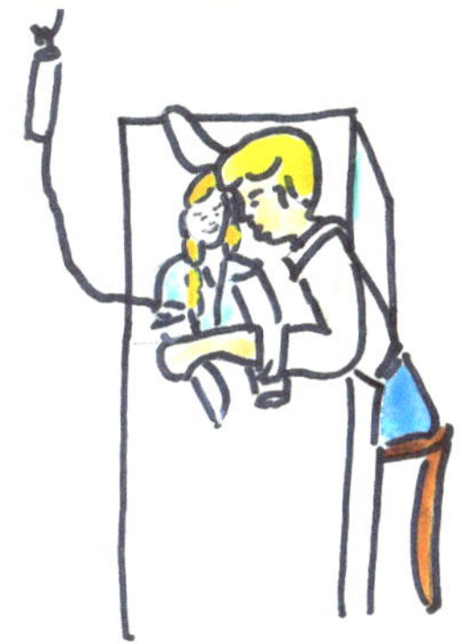

My father was working for the railroad. He worked seven days a week, sixteen hours a day. In 1943, the railroad was very important for the war effort. Most of the young men had gone to war; railroad men were deferred from the military, and they worked double shifts to keep the trains running. My father's workday was from eight o'clock in the morning until twelve o'clock at midnight. The only time he could visit me was before eight in the morning or after midnight. He would come to see me on his way home from work at midnight. I looked forward to seeing him every evening. I would not go to sleep until he came. The doctor worried that his visits disrupted my sleep. He asked my father to stop visiting me at midnight. I was furious I needed to see him. How could he expect me to sleep until my father came? The doctor could not make me go to sleep before he came, no matter how much medicine he gave me. Finally, he told my father he should probably come back and visit me on his way home from work. I would fall asleep in a few minutes with my father by my bed.

I started getting better. I was awake more. I enjoyed company. The volunteers were my friends. They would talk to me, play games with me, and read stories. My favorite thing was when my mother would come and sing to me about little girls, faraway places, lullabies, and love songs.

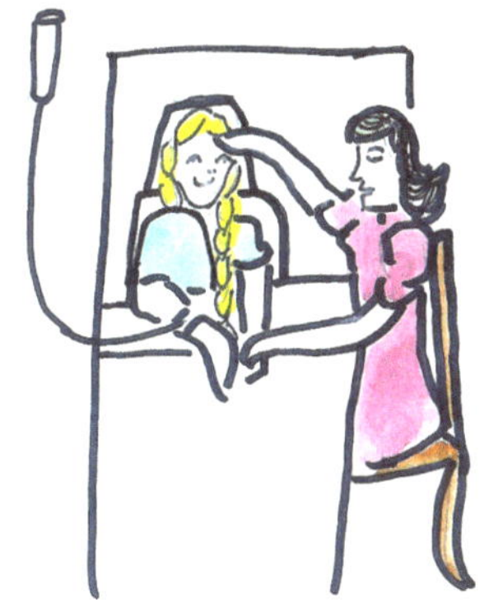

Once in a while, Tyke and my cousins would come to visit me. They couldn't come in my room because they might bring infections that would make me sick again. There was a little porch outside my window, and the kids would come there and talk to me. Alan, my cousin, had broken his arm before I broke mine. He didn't have to stay in the hospital. I remember asking him how come he didn't have to stay in the hospital, and he told me he had a better doctor.

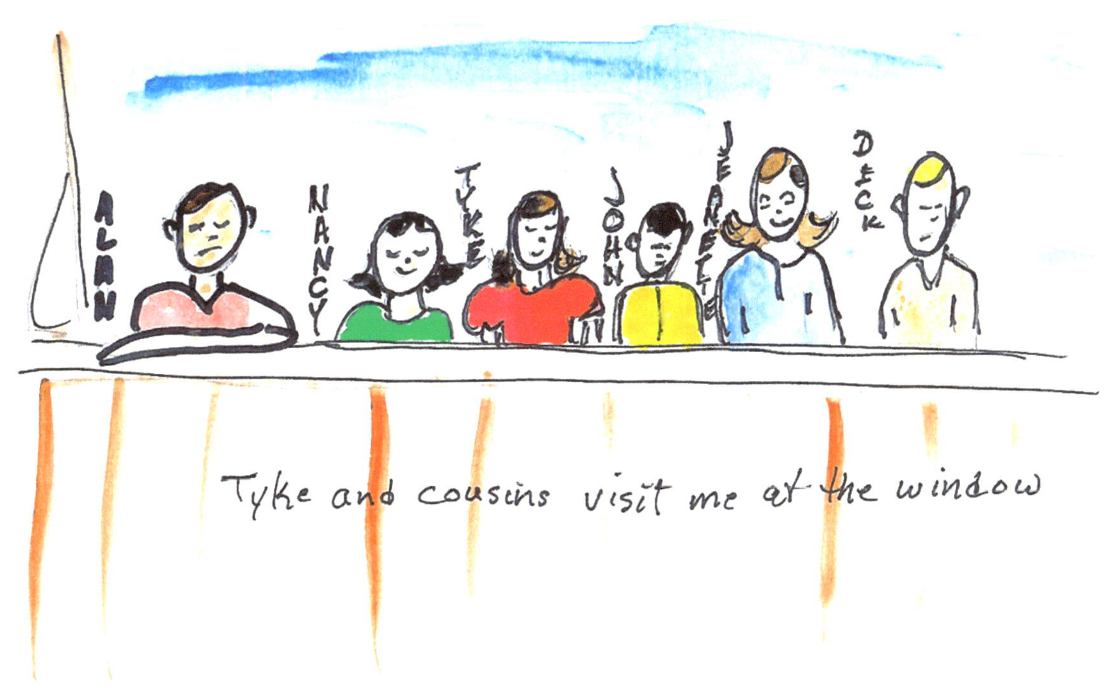

Tyke and cousins visit me at the window

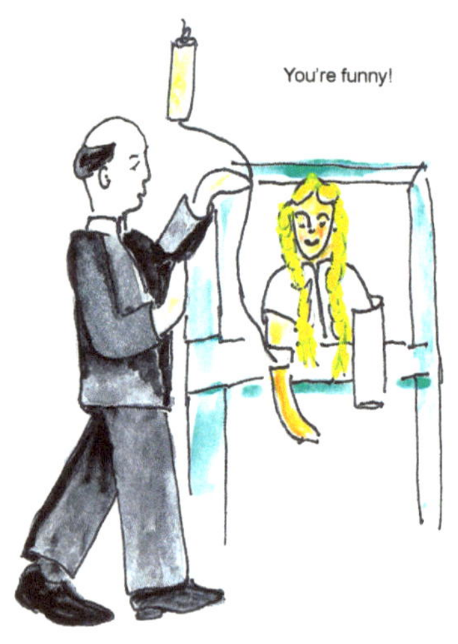

One of the people who came to visit me often was Fr. McGoldrick. He was the priest for the Catholic Church in Portola. He had given me the last rites when I was very ill. When I asked him what *last rites* were, he told me it was my first communion. We became friends. I used to love to have him come and see me because he would tell stories and sing songs about Ireland. He spoke with an Irish accent; he made me laugh when he told jokes and stories. I couldn't understand much of what he said because of his accent.

I liked having people around to keep me company. I wasn't feeling as bad. I was getting restless. I was tired of lying down. Dr. McKnight told my parents it was time to let me know I had one arm. I had no idea that my arm was not in the cast that had been on the bed ever since the amputation. I could feel my hand and my elbow, and I could feel my fingers move. Occasionally, I would get sharp pains in my fingers or my elbow in my broken arm. I asked my mother to scratch my arm in the cast because it was itchy. She scratched the itchy spot with a knitting needle every time I asked her to.

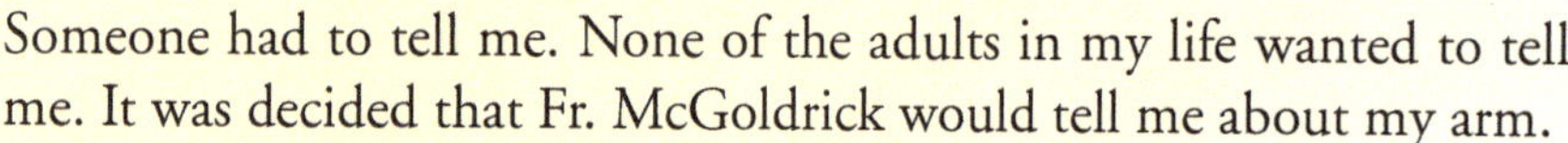

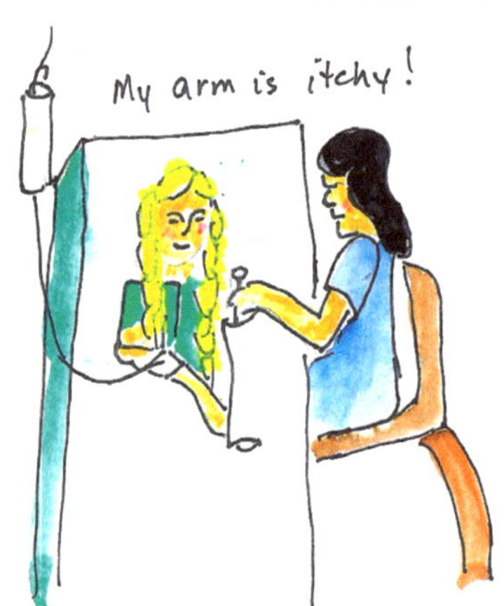

Someone had to tell me. None of the adults in my life wanted to tell me. It was decided that Fr. McGoldrick would tell me about my arm.

The truth will out!

Chapter 6

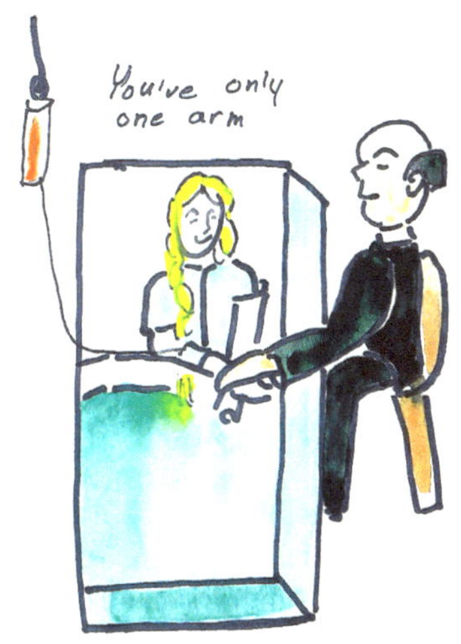

There was a soft knock at the door, and Fr. McGoldrick entered my room. I knew something was wrong; he was very serious, he wasn't telling jokes, and he wasn't laughing or singing. He sat next to my bed and said, "How are you this fine morning?" He took my hand in his hand and added, "Are you okay?" I replied, "What's the matter?" I knew something was wrong because he looked so serious. He told me I had to be very brave and not to cry. I asked him what was wrong. He said everything was fine. I was getting better, and I would soon be going home. "But the one thing you need to know, missy, before you go, is that you've only one arm. Now, don't be crying about it. Do you understand, lassie?" I remember trying to figure out what he was talking about, but I promised I would not cry. I was a big girl. I was almost eight years old. I was not a crybaby!

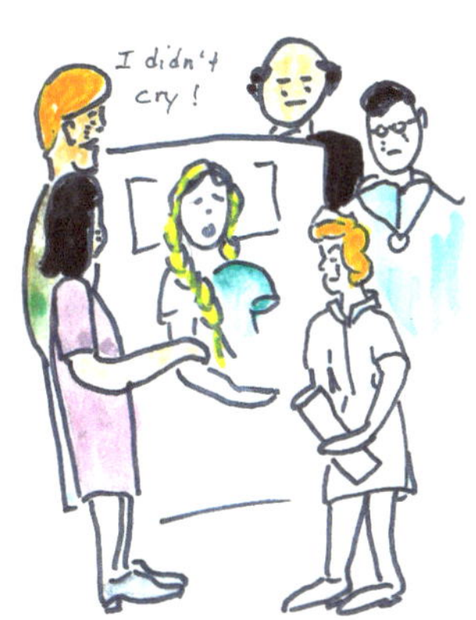

Fr. McGoldrick stood up and opened the door. I was still trying to understand what was happening when the nurse, the doctor, and my parents came into the room. They gathered round my bed as the nurse took away the cast. "What did he say? What was he trying to tell me? How can they take the cast away? He said you've only one arm. Oh my god! I have only one arm. I cannot cry. I promised."

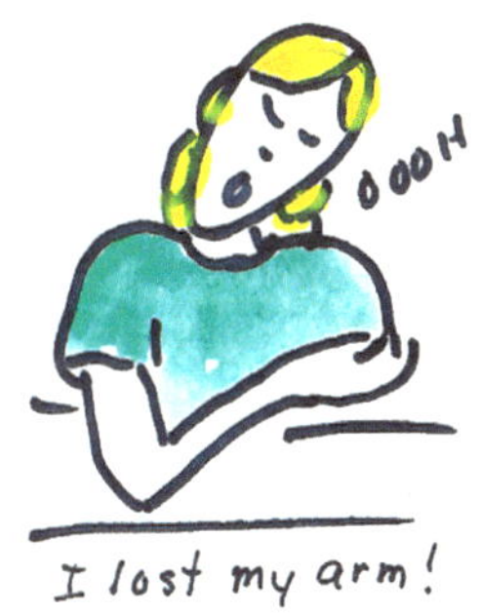

When they removed the cast, my whole left side felt cold and damp. I tried to look at my left side. I wanted to see my arm or what was left of my arm. There was nothing there. There was *nothing* there. I couldn't breathe. My head was pounding. I thought I was going to throw up. I felt hot and sweaty. It was like going too fast in a car over a big bump you feel like your stomach had dropped. I didn't want anybody to know that I was scared. I was not a crybaby. I was so scared! I said I wouldn't cry, and I didn't cry. I was horrified!

I had no idea that my arm was not in the cast that had been on the bed ever since the operation to fix my arm. I could feel my hand and my elbow, and I could feel my fingers move. Occasionally, I would get sharp pains in my fingers or my elbow in my arm in the cast. I remember asking my mother to scratch my arm in the cast because it was itchy. I knew my broken arm was in that cast.

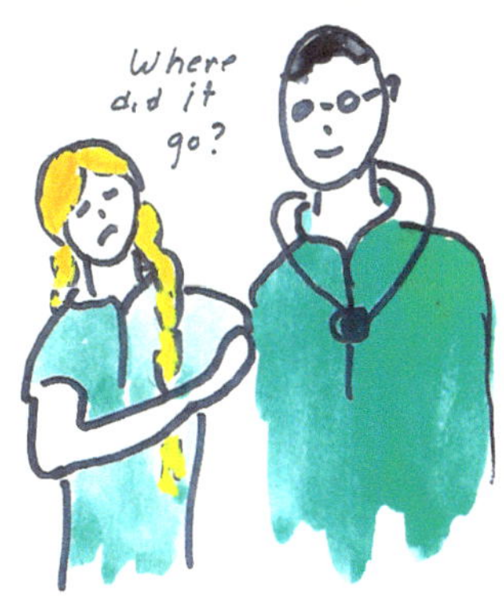

I looked at Mom and asked her what had happened. She said I had lost my arm. I said, "What happened? How can I lose my arm?" I looked at Dr. McKnight. "How did I lose my arm? Where did it go? What happened to me? Why didn't my arm get better? When the cast comes off of a broken arm, it is supposed to be all better." I looked at my parents; they were both crying. The nurse was gone; she had taken the cast out of the room. Fr. McGoldrick was crying. Dr. McKnight came very close to me, and he said I didn't lose my arm because it was broken. I lost my arm because of a very serious infection. I asked him again, "How can I lose my arm? Where did it go?" He answered, "Your arm had to be amputated so that you wouldn't die from the infection." I asked what *amputated* meant. He said it meant that he had to cut my arm off so I could get well. I was afraid to ask him what he had done with my arm.

Everybody in the room was crying except me.

Chapter 7

The shock of learning I had only one arm didn't last long because I was able to sit up in bed. It felt very good to sit up. I could draw pictures, use colored crayons, and look straight at people—not up at them. I couldn't sit up very long because I would tire quickly. The drawing and coloring was fun, but I soon wanted to do everything. I told my mother that when I got home, I would have to be able to tie my shoes. She said no. She would get me buckle shoes. I said, "I don't want buckle shoes." I had learned how to tie my shoes before I got hurt. I wanted to tie shoes. After some discussion, Mom said, "All right, I'll get you shoes to tie." She bought me a brand-new pair of tie shoes. It took me about a week to figure out how to tie the shoes with one hand. No one at the hospital thought I would be able to tie shoes. I felt very good about myself when I finally could tie my own shoes.

This is hard!

I can do it!

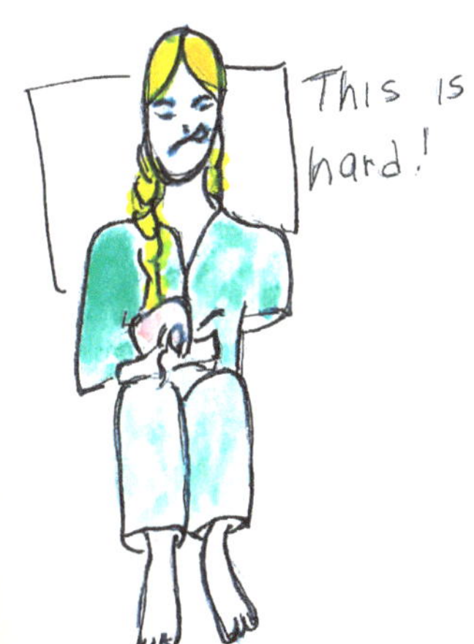

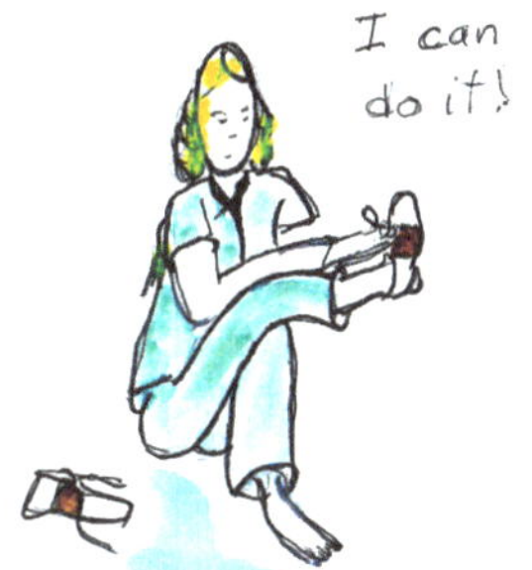

Now that I could tie my shoes, I put them on every morning. I asked every morning if I could walk around my room. The nurses said no. When the doctor came to see me, I told him I wanted to walk around my room. He said I was too weak even to stand up. I was very disappointed. I did not believe that I could not walk. He made sure that there was always a volunteer with me so that I would not get out of bed and try to walk home by myself. He acted like me walking home was kind of a joke, but he meant it.

I felt frustrated and impatient because they would not let me walk. I told Mom I needed a new project. I decided I needed to learn how to cut paper with one hand. Mom brought magazines and paper dolls for me to cut. She bought me some small sharp scissors, and we started practicing cutting. Cutting was harder than tying shoes. It took awhile to figure out how to hold things in order to cut straight lines. I figured out if I held the paper with my knees, I could cut. It wasn't long before I started cutting out paper dolls. The paper dolls were not perfect, but I felt good about being able to do it.

Cutting is harder than tying shoes!

The next problem we had was about my hair. Because I had to lie on my back for weeks, the hair at the back of my head was one big mat. While I had been comatose, I constantly moved my head back and forth causing it to snarl. My mother said we should cut my hair. I said, "No, I do not want my hair cut." She said, "It will hurt to comb out the snarl. It is a very big tangled mess of hair. It will hurt a lot to comb it out." I said, "I don't care how much it hurts. I want long hair." My mother really didn't want to untangle my hair with a comb because she knew it would be very painful for me. She went to visit the hair dresser at a little shop in town. She asked her if there was any way or anything she could put on my hair so it wouldn't hurt so badly when she combed it out. The hair dresser suggested she use witch hazel. She warned my mother that witch hazel did not smell good. She gave Mom the witch hazel. Mom started on my hair the next day. The hair dresser was right; it didn't smell good. It took about a week of careful combing, and eventually, the snarl was out. My hair looked like a dirty mop and smelled worse, but it was still on my head.

Sorry!
Ouch!
Witch Hazel

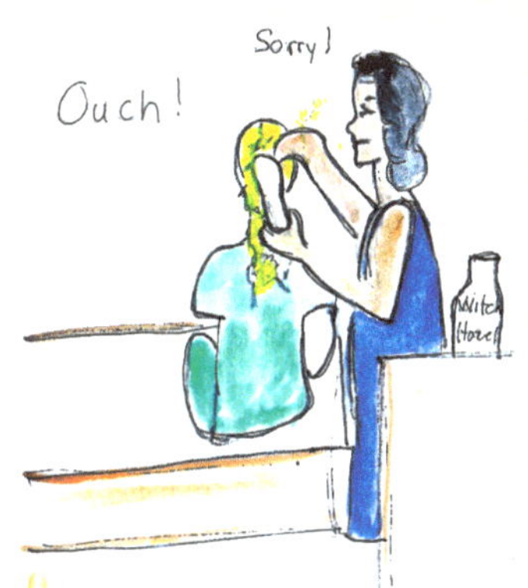

I was feeling pretty good. The doctor was starting to talk about when I would go home. I had been doing somersaults—standing on my head, putting my feet flat on the bed pretending to walk, and doing everything a person can possibly do on a bed without falling out of it. I told the doctor it was time for me to walk. He said, "Not yet. You cannot walk, you are not strong enough, and your legs will not hold your body up." I told him I was sure I could walk because my legs and my feet were fine.

See! My feet are fine.

I can't walk!

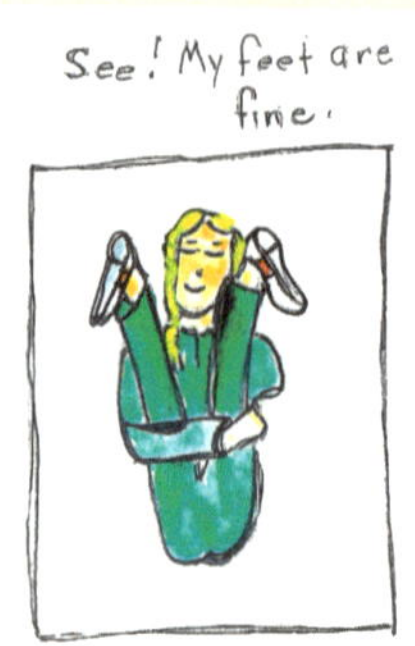

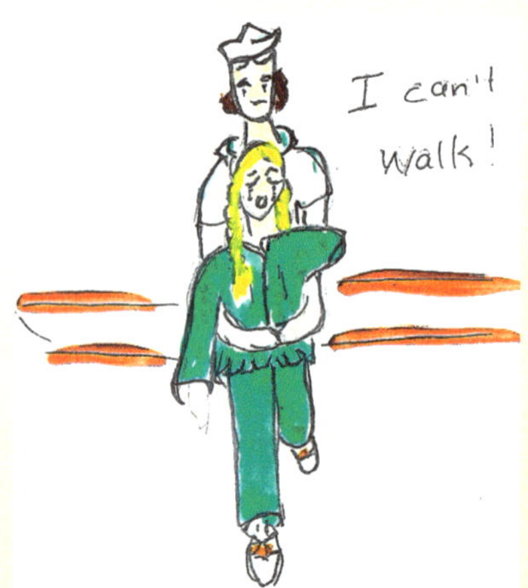

Later, when my favorite nurse came in to check on me, I asked her to help me walk. She told me that I probably couldn't stand up by myself. I told her that I felt very strong, and I was sure I could do it if she would help me. She said, "Okay, I will help you to walk to the door, if you promise to let me hold you." I said, "Okay." She put my shoes on my feet. I tied them. She helped me out of the bed. Holding on to my waist, standing behind me, she said, "Okay walk." I took my first step, and I couldn't hold myself up. She helped me to the door, pretty much carrying me all the way, and then helped me back into bed. I was devastated. I couldn't believe that I could not walk. My feet were fine. My legs were fine. But I couldn't walk. They were all right, and I was all wrong. I was so mad and disappointed. It wasn't fair. I cried like a baby. I couldn't stop crying. The nurse sat on the bed with both her arms around me. She told me that everything would be fine—my legs were fine, and my feet were fine. She said all I needed to do was get stronger. She told me I didn't need to worry. In a week or two I'd be moving around just fine. She said, "You may cry if you want to." I cried for a long time while she held me close to her. Finally, I stopped, we hugged each other, and I told her I was okay. "I don't need to cry anymore. Please don't tell anyone I cried." She said, "You have good reason to cry. It's okay, but I will keep your secret. I'll be back to see you in a little while." It was the first time I dared to let myself cry. I didn't want anyone to know that having an arm amputated was a terrible thing.

It is not Fair!

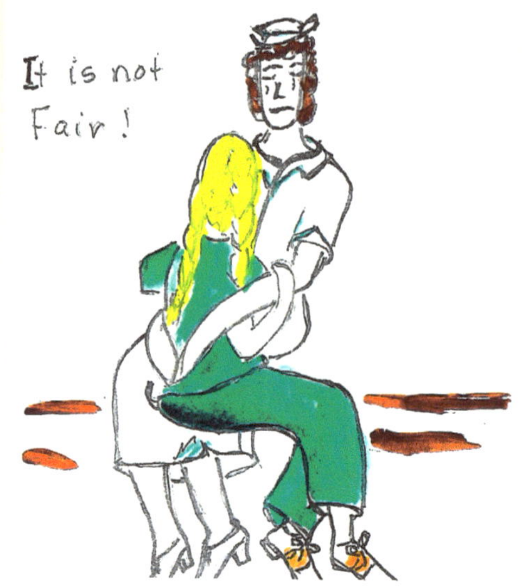

The next day, Dr. McKnight told me I would be going home soon. I hadn't been eating very well. My going-away gift from Dr. McKnight was that I could have anything I wanted to eat for my last meal. They had been trying to give me milk shakes, homemade ice cream, hot chocolate, and anything else they thought I might like. I didn't like anything they gave me to eat. For my last meal at the hospital, I chose fried chicken with mashed potatoes and gravy, fresh peas, and salad. He asked me what I wanted for dessert, and I said strawberry shortcake with fresh strawberries. By that time, it was the end of September. The strawberry season was over in our part of the state. Dr. McKnight had a friend who lived in Los Angeles. He asked him to fly some fresh strawberries from the Imperial Valley to Reno, Nevada. The strawberries were delivered to Portola in time for my last dinner. My father and Dr. McKnight came to sit with me while I ate that very special dinner. I could not eat the chicken. I could not eat the potatoes and gravy. I could not eat the peas nor the salad. I did eat the strawberry shortcake. My father and Dr. McKnight ate the rest of my dinner. Everybody was happy.

Soon after the walking practice and the special dinner, I was able to go home. I was unable to walk; I had lost half my body weight in a month. I looked a lot like the refugees from the concentration camps in Germany. My arm would not heal. The infection was no longer a danger to my life, but the wound would not heal. The affected tissue continued to produce a residue, which drained from the stump of my arm. The skin would heal over the wound. When the wound would close, my arm would become very painful, like a toothache from the pressure. When this happened, the doctor would lance the skin and allow it to drain. This was not a satisfactory situation. I also had a problem sitting. I had received very large hypodermic injections of penicillin in my hips. I received a shot every hour for weeks. I was so thin, and there was so little muscle that it was painful to sit in a regular chair. I was still wearing a bandage on my arm—it was big, it had to be changed by the doctor every day, and all the skin that had been taped was red and sore. It felt like a burn when the tape was taken off so they could replace the bandage. I had to go to the hospital every day to have my bandage changed. I was weak and underweight. In August before I got hurt, I weighed sixty-five pounds. When I came home from the hospital a month later, I weighed thirty pounds. The doctor prepared a special tonic to help me gain strength and improve my weight. It was the worst tasting stuff I have ever consumed. The first few days, I threw it up every time they gave it to me. It was awful. In time I was able to keep it down, but it never tasted any better. I was still a sick kid, but I was so glad to be home.

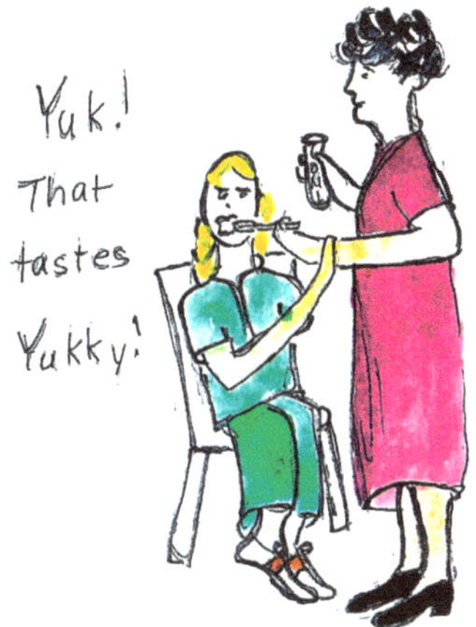

The hard work begins!

Chapter 8

I like doing dishes

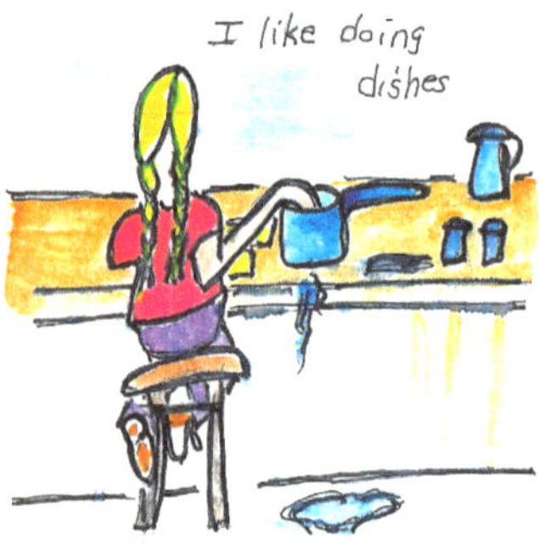

Now that I was home, it was time to become part of the family again. The first order of business was to start walking. I began by walking around things, holding on to something so I wouldn't fall. My legs were so weak that if I didn't hang on to something, they just stopped holding me up. At first I couldn't go very far because I was weak and would get tired. Little by little I gained strength enough to walk across the room with help. That was a great milestone. My father or my sister or someone would help me get to the sink so I could wash dishes. I would sit on a high stool and play in the water until the dishes were clean. I felt really good about helping Mom with the dishes, and it was fun playing in the water.

My sister, Tyke, and I played paper dolls. We sat on the floor, and she would have some dolls, and I would have some, and we would create social situations with our paper dolls. I loved playing with her. Tyke was my best friend and only playmate.

Paper

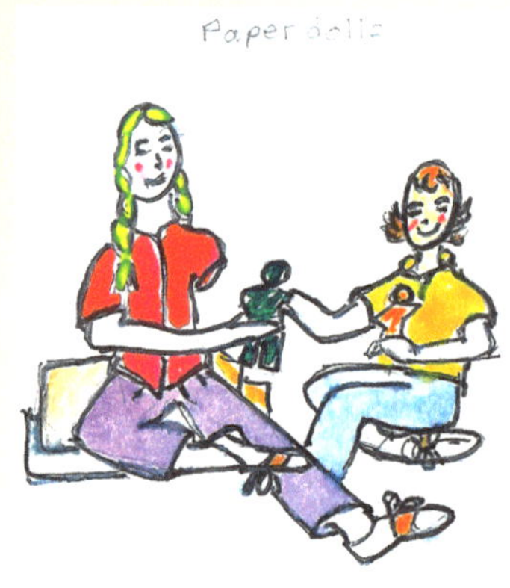

The people in Portola knew I had been hurt. They knew that I was very underweight and weak. Many of them had taken care of me in the hospital as volunteers. Everybody seemed to want to help us. This was during World War II when many food products were rationed. People in town brought ration stamps or eggs, fruits, vegetables, and other foodstuffs they thought I might need. Our family will never forget how wonderful the people in Portola were to us.

May I hold it?

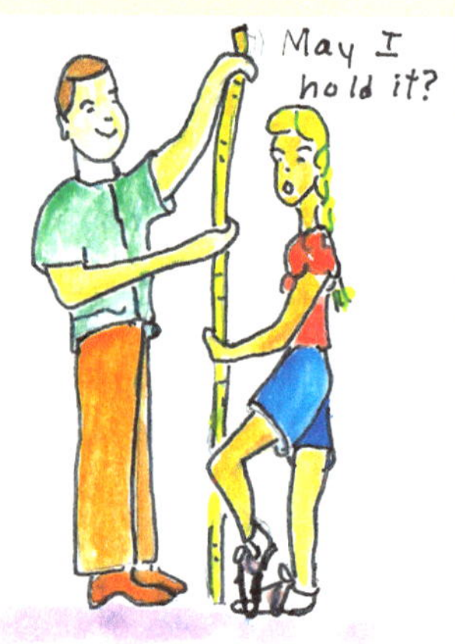

Every day I got stronger. I was walking around the house with a little help. I could take several steps by myself. I decided it was time to go outside. My mother said I could go, but she would help me out, and she would watch me. I didn't really think I needed to be watched, but I didn't argue. I remember we walked out across the front porch and down the step to the ground. It'd been almost two months since I had been outside with my feet on the ground. It was exhilarating. There were children outside who came over to talk to me. After we talked for a while, I sat down. They were playing with a bamboo pole. It was a long pole probably four or five feet long. While I was sitting on the step, my mother went back into the house. The boy holding the bamboo pole came over to talk to me. I asked him if I wanted to hold the pole. I stood up, and he handed it to me. I held it in my hand, and he let go. It was so heavy I couldn't hold it up. I put my leg next to the pole to balance it. Something stung my leg, and I dropped the bamboo pole. I cried out with pain. Everyone rushed to see what had happened.

A bee stung my leg!

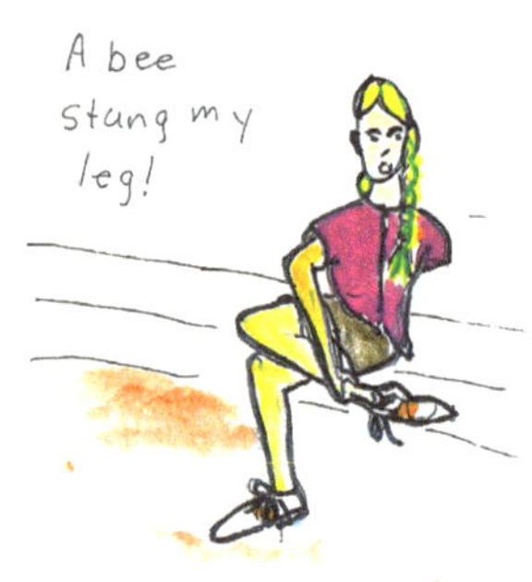

My mother came running out of the house with a worried look on her face. She asked me why I had cried out. I looked down at my leg where it had touched the pole. There was a bee on my leg; it had stung me. My leg began to swell almost immediately after the sting.

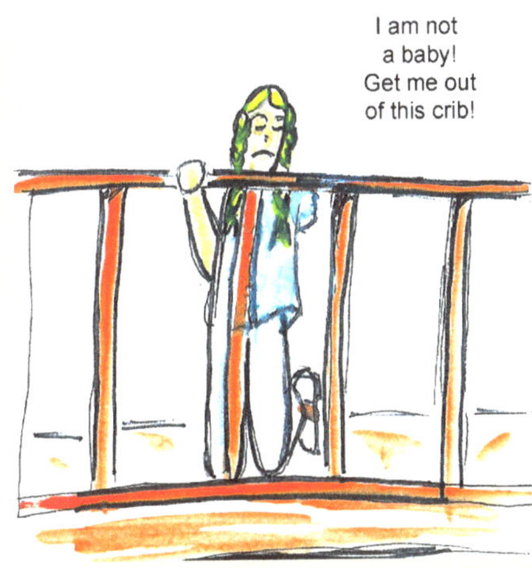

Mom took me to the hospital. When I got to the hospital, the doctor took one look at my leg and admitted me into the hospital for observation. The nurse put me in a crib with four sides up. I was very upset. I told her the doctor would be angry because I was not a baby. I did not want to be in a crib. I did not want to stay there. When Dr. McKnight came to see me, he agreed I did not belong in a crib. He told the nurse that I was to be moved to a regular sized bed as soon as possible. I felt a lot better.

I asked the doctor why I had to stay in the hospital for just a bee sting. He told me that I had a bad reaction to the sting, probably because my body was still fighting off the effects of the gangrene infection. He said I shouldn't worry or be afraid. He told my parents that I should be able to do anything I want to do. If I got hurt, like a bee sting, we would deal with it like any other child. After a day in the hospital, I was fine, and they sent me home. My leg was still sore and red, but the swelling had gone down.

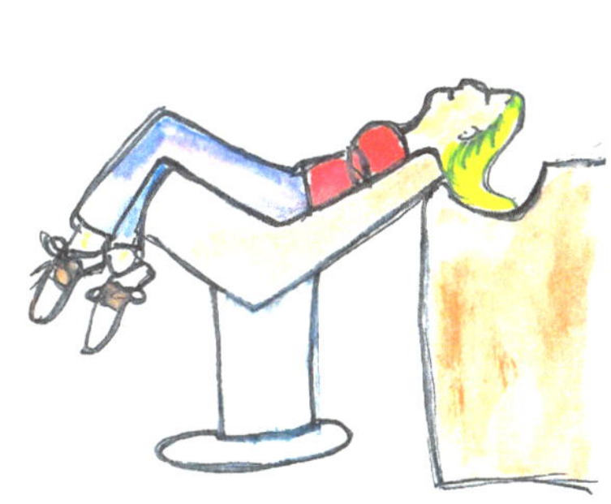

The day after I came home from the hospital, recovering from my bee sting, my mother said she could not stand another day looking at and smelling my hair. The witch hazel had helped to get the snarls out of my hair. It had not been washed in almost two months. My mother was afraid of getting my bandage wet. She asked a hair dresser if she thought she could wash my hair safely. She said she could, and she did. She wrapped a rubber sheet all around my bandage. Then she had me hang my head back over the basin while she washed my hair. My sticky, dirty blonde hair became bright, shiny, and silky. My mother, my father, and I were delighted. I smelled much better. I felt great with clean hair. My grandma Souza came on the train from Sacramento to our house in Portola the day before I got my hair washed. Mom thought the baby would be born soon. Grandma came to Portola to take Tyke home with her while Mom went to the hospital to have the baby. Grandma went home with Tyke the day I got my hair washed.

The day after my hair was washed, my baby brother arrived. His name was Donald Leonard Tibbedeaux Jr. It was October 2, 1943. My father and I were very excited! He took me to the greasy spoon—that was the nickname for a little restaurant down by the train depot in Portola. Uncle Alfred and Uncle Adrian, my father's brothers, joined us for a major celebration. We toasted to the new baby. We toasted that I was home and getting better, and we toasted to Mom being well and happy. Everyone in the restaurant toasted to us. They all wished us well.

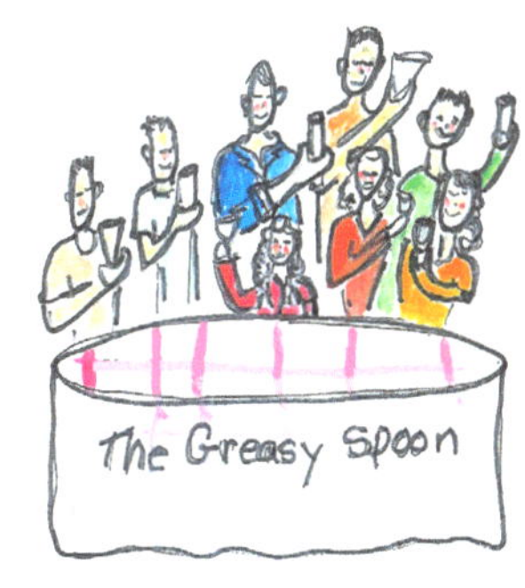

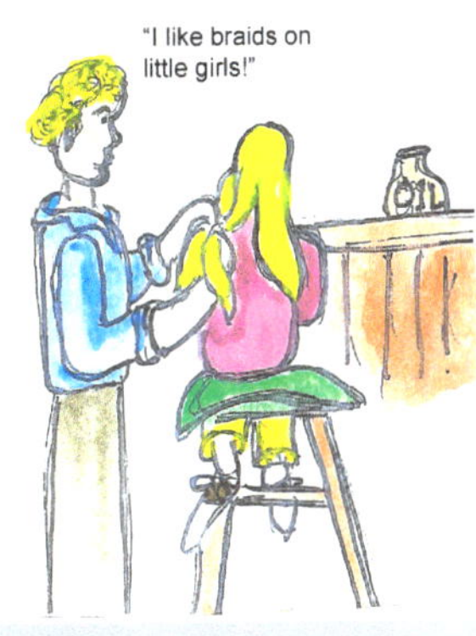

The next day, my father had to comb my hair to take me to see Mom at the hospital. As I said, my hair hadn't been washed in almost two months, so it was very silky and slippery. My father thought he should braid my hair. He said he liked little girls with braids. That was fine with me. As he tried to braid my hair, it kept slipping out of the braids, so he got hair oil. He put enough on my hair so that it didn't slip anymore. In fact, it stuck together pretty effectively. When we got to the hospital to see Mom and the baby, my mother was horrified. All she could see was greasy, smelly hair. She said, "What did you do to her hair?" My father answered, "I put hair oil on it so I could braid it. I think it looks fine." We all laughed.

It was a very happy event—I was getting better, the baby had arrived, and he was healthy. Mom was feeling good and would come home in a few days. My sister would come home, and our family would all be together—happy, healthy, and well.

New beginnings!

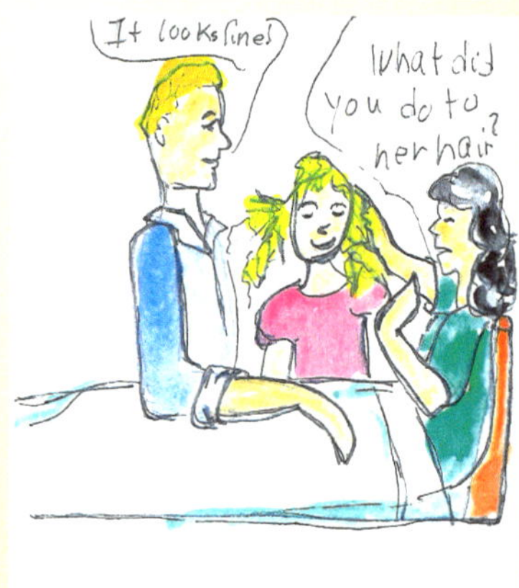

Chapter 9

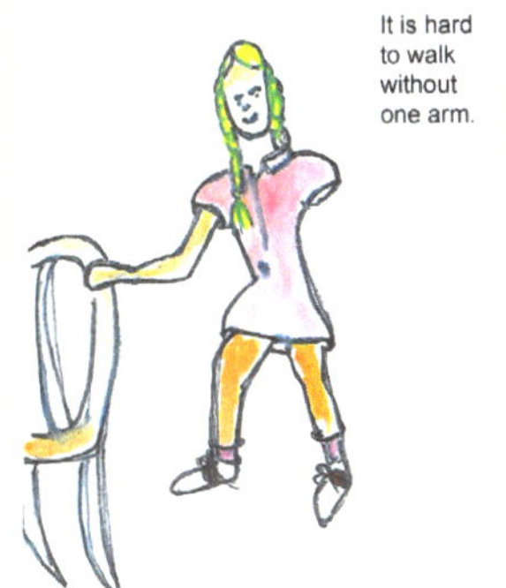

Tyke returned home from Grandma's house about the middle of October. School had already started. Tyke would begin second grade a few weeks late. I wanted to go to school too. The doctor said I was not well enough. The infection was still draining out of my arm. I had to have my bandage changed daily. I needed to get stronger, and I needed to improve my balance. When I finally started to walk independently, it became clear that learning to walk was a more complicated process than any of us understood. Because I had lost my arm, my bilateral movement was off center. I would try to walk a straight line. I would lean to the left then to the right to get where I needed to go. The doctor said maybe ballet dancing would help me with my balance.

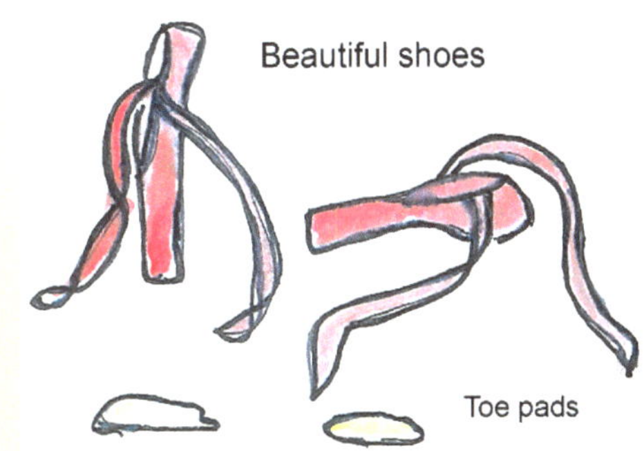

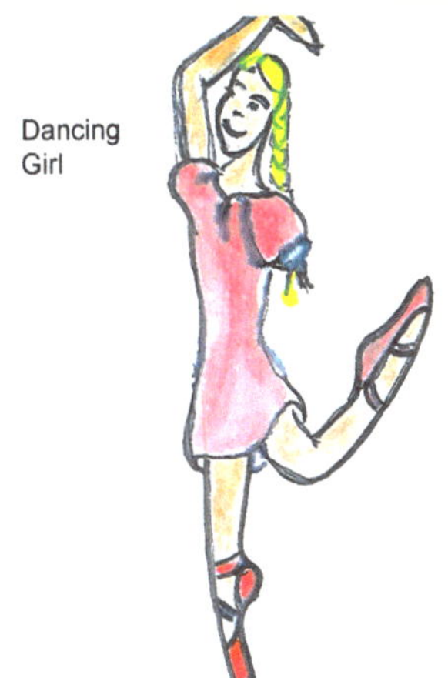

There was no dance school in Portola. My mother ordered a pair of hard toe ballet slippers from the Sears catalog for me. I loved them. They were pink satin with long pink satin tie ribbons. I practiced walking and dancing every day. The ballet slippers were hard to walk in. I wore little lamb's wool pads to protect my toes, but they still got sore. It felt good to stand straight and tall, to take small steps, holding my head as high as I could with my arm arched over my head. Sometimes I would hold on to the side of a kitchen chair and point my toes first one leg and then the other as far forward or back as I could while standing as straight as I could. I danced almost every day until I outgrew the shoes. I don't know how much they helped with my balance, but they were wonderful for my self-esteem.

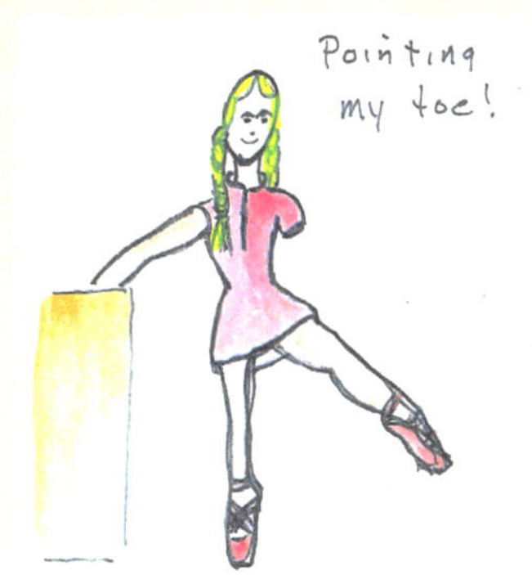

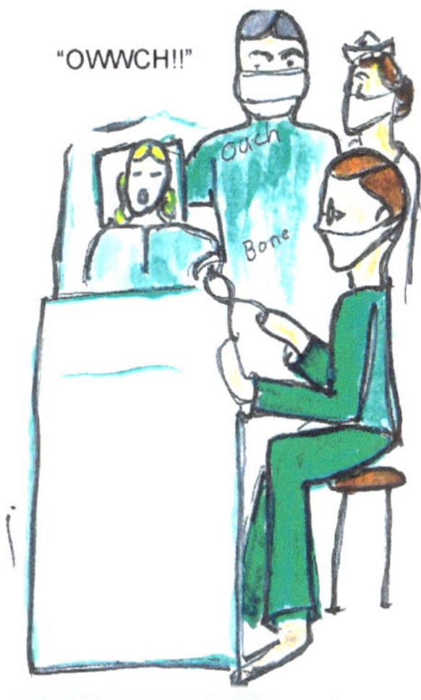

By November, my arm had not improved; the wound would not heal. The skin was healing, but the infection was still draining. When the wound would close, pressure would build under the skin, and my arm would throb like a toothache. The doctor thought that perhaps the bone had not been cut short enough. He thought that maybe that was why the skin would heal, but the drainage would not stop. So it was decided that they would have to take a small portion from the bottom of the bone in my arm. They gave me a local anesthetic and then used a tool that looked like a pair of pliers with a sharp, flat tip for cutting or snipping. They snipped off the tip of the bone. It felt like it would feel if they used that tool on my tooth without pain killer. It felt very strange, like an electric shock. It jarred my whole body. I screamed, but I did not cry.

That operation did not work. Within a day or two, the skin had grown over the stump of my arm again. Dr. McKnight and his colleagues were puzzled. My arm would not heal until they could stop the drainage from the infection. They did not understand why it was still draining. I was getting better and stronger every day, but obviously, my arm had not healed. Dr. McKnight contacted Stanford Hospital & Clinics in San Francisco. He consulted with Dr. King, the head of orthopedic surgery at Stanford. Dr. King wanted to examine the wound.

He expected that infection was causing the drainage. He thought additional surgery would be necessary to rid the wound of infection and stop the problem. He was also very interested in the penicillin test case for gas gangrene. The problem was that the hospital was full and would take some time to arrange for me to go there.

Dr. McKnight sent all my records to Stanford hospital for Dr. King to review. It was arranged for me to go to San Francisco and be examined by Dr. King shortly after the first of the year. Penicillin was a miracle drug; it was saving lives that historically would have been lost. Every medical facility in the country wanted to learn about penicillin. Stanford was a teaching hospital. Learning about the effects of this new drug on gas gangrene was a rare and important event in medical history.

New clothes!

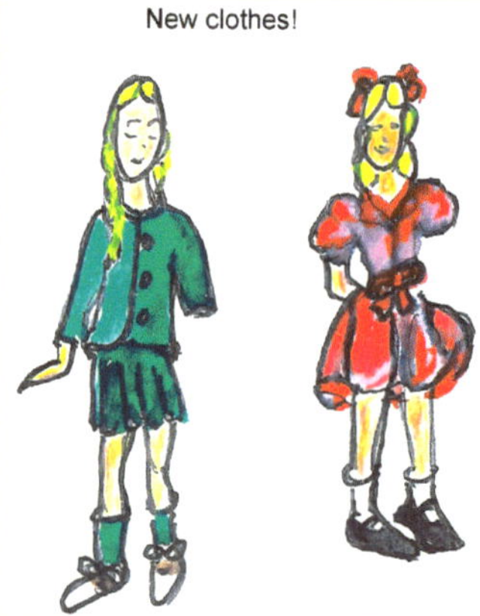

We could hardly believe it! Dad, Mom, and I were going to the city! We had to get ready! Mom said Dad's suit would be fine. Mom had a nice suit she could wear and a dressy dress to wear to dinner, but I had nothing to wear. All my clothes were too short. I exclaimed, "Oh no! I can't go!" Mom and Daddy started to laugh. "You're the reason we are going, silly. I said, "I cannot go without clothes!" Mom put her arms around me and said, "I will make you a suit for traveling and a party dress in case you need one." I was so excited. I had never been to a really big city. I knew that it was a very important trip because Daddy was taking off from work to come and be with Mom and me.

San Francisco was a major seaport city on the Pacific coast. In 1944, servicemen were everywhere. Some were coming back from fighting in the war in the Pacific. Some were leaving to go fight in the Pacific. Hotel rooms were very hard to get. Every kind of entertainment was sold out almost before the production began. When I went to San Francisco in 1944, Dr. McKnight, my parents, and I stayed at a beautiful hotel. Dr. King had arranged to make our stay in San Francisco a memorable and pleasant experience. Our hotel suite included two bedrooms and a sitting room. Two officers (I think they were soldiers in the army) and their wives were still in our rooms when we got there. The men were going to war, and their wives were sadly saying good-bye. They welcomed us into the rooms. They asked if we were on vacation. Mom told them I was a test case for penicillin. I was having surgery so my wound would heal. The two couples wished me well. We wished them well because they were going to war. Then we said good-bye, and they left.

That night, we met Dr. King and his wife and Dr. McKnight for dinner at a very nice restaurant. After dinner, we went to the Follies. It was the first time I had gone to a show where all the people in the show sang and danced and told jokes. We laughed, clapped our hands, and cheered. We had a wonderful time.

"Oh! No! The clothes fell out of the suitcase!"

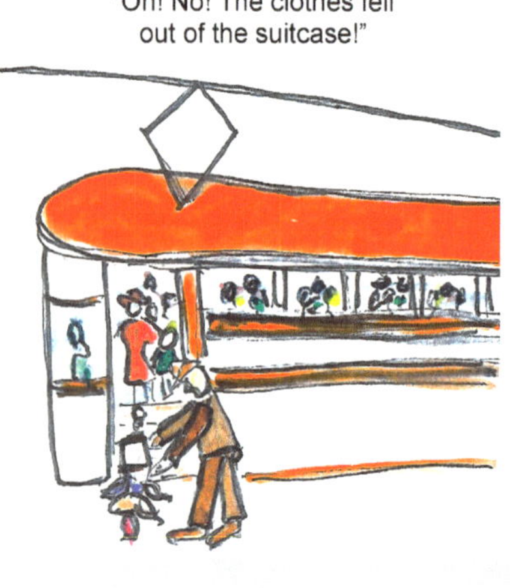

The next morning, we got up, dressed, packed our suitcase, and ate breakfast in the hotel dining room. Then we left the hotel and went to the streetcar stop to go to Stanford-Lane Hospital. The hospital was huge. It was a city block big and about ten stories high. We went to the hospital the morning after our wonderful party. My parents and I took a streetcar to the hospital. It was a beautiful day, and we were excited to be in the city. We brought our suitcase because Mom and Dad were going to the train after I was admitted into the hospital. Everything was great until the suitcase opened as we were getting on the streetcar. Clothes fell out of the suitcase down the steps into the street. Daddy had to gather up all the socks, underwear, and everything else we had packed. I started to laugh. Mom was smiling. "That is not funny, Yvonne." Daddy said he wished we had left the suitcase home.

"It is NOT funny!"

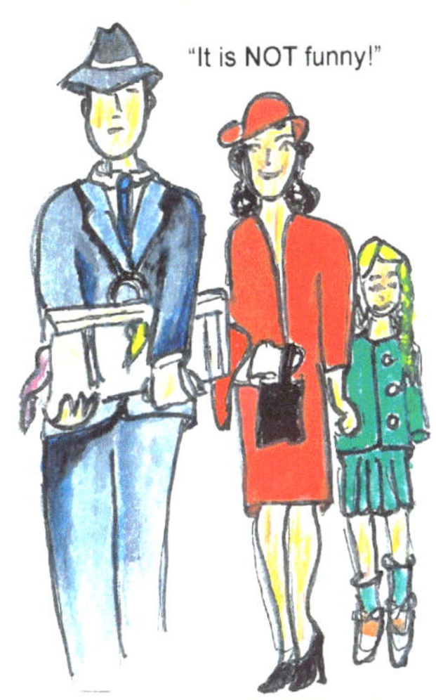

The people at the desk at the hospital were expecting me. A nurse took us to the children's ward where my bed was located. The doctors met us there in a little meeting room and explained that I would have to have x-rays and all kinds of tests. Daddy asked how long I would need to stay in the hospital in San Francisco. The doctor said until the tests were done. "We don't know how long that will take. After the tests are completed, we will operate to remove the cause of the draining. If we are successful, she should be able to go home by the end of this month." When the wound in my arm stopped draining, I would be all better. After the doctors explained to us what was going to happen, they shook hands with my dad and told my parents they would take good care of me, and they wished them a safe trip home. Then the doctor looked at me and said, "I'll see you tomorrow, young lady." After the doctors left, Mom helped me put on the pj's that were on my bed. The pajamas were too big. Mom said, "Better too big than too small." And we both laughed. My parents said it was time for them to go because the train was leaving soon. Daddy had to work, and Mom had to take care of Donnie and Tyke. Mom would visit me every week, and she would make a special trip to be with me when I had the surgery. She would come down on the train, leave Donnie and Tyke in Sacramento with Grandma, and come to the hospital and see me. They hugged me, told me that I would be fine and to remember that this surgery would heal the wound in my arm and make me well again. Then they kissed me good-bye, and they left.

Mom will visit
every week

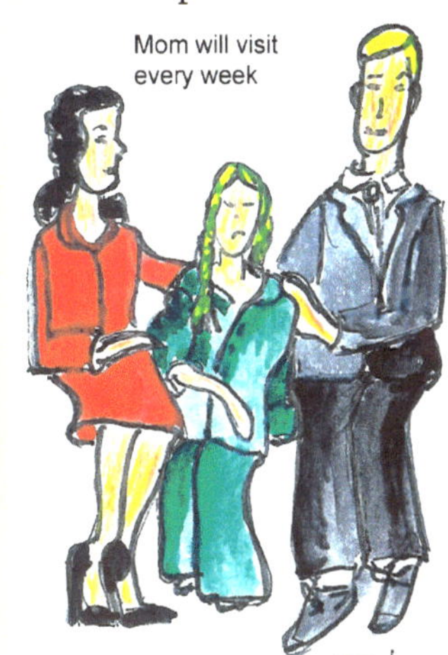

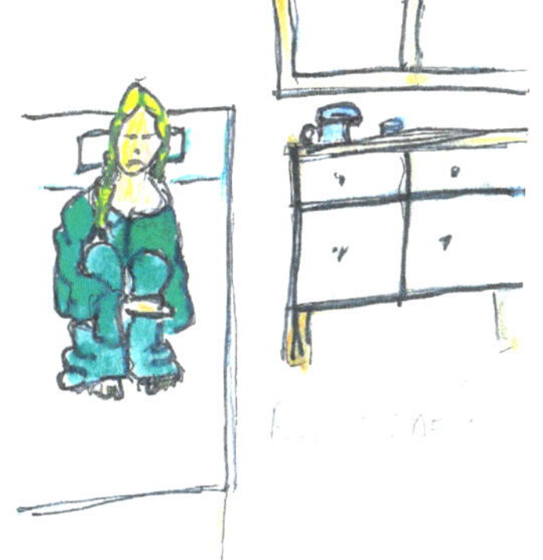

San Francisco was a very long way from Portola. It took us twelve hours on the train to get here. There were different areas on different floors of this hospital that were bigger than the whole hospital in Portola. The children's ward was bigger than Portola hospital. I didn't know anyone here, and no one knew me. I sat on my bed in a little glass cubicle with curtains hung all around so I couldn't see out, and no one could see in. I was very alone. I could hear people moving around and talking outside of my cubicle. So after a while, I decided to get off the bed and see what was on the other side of my curtain.

When I peeked out of my curtain, I saw a long room with lots of little cubicles. Some of the cubicles had the curtain pulled back. There were children in those cubicles. I wanted to explore the whole room, but I was afraid to leave my cubicle until I was sure that the doctor and nurses knew I was there. I opened my curtain so I could sit on the bed and look out.

Peeking
around
the
curtain

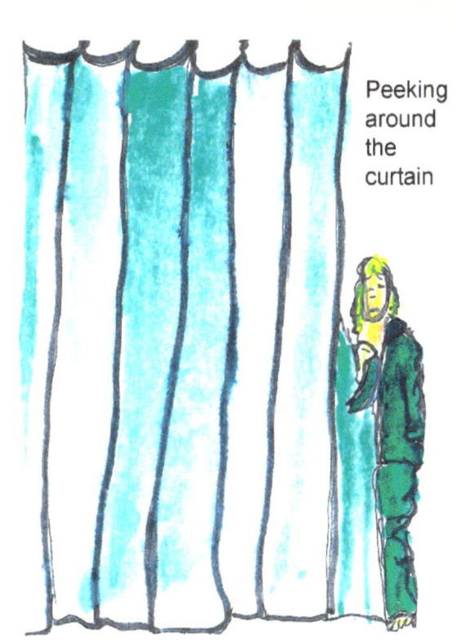

After a very short time, the biggest darkest, jolliest lady I had ever seen came into my cubicle and said, "My goodness! What a beautiful little girl we have staying with us." I asked if she was Mammy from *Gone with the Wind*. She laughed and said, "Nobody ever called me a movie star before. Wouldn't that be something?" She asked me if I wanted to just sit there all day or come and help her. I told her I

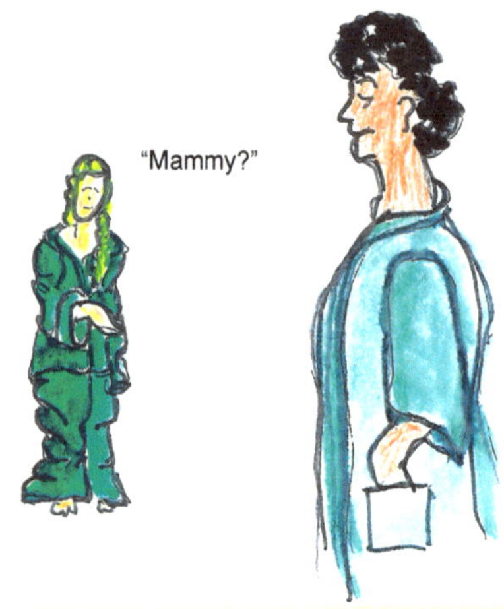

would like to help her. "What can I do?" She said she had to deliver water to all the bed tables in our ward. She said she sure could use someone to take the water from the cart to the tables. I told her, "I could do that." She said, "Okay, come along." I had a job. I was so happy that she needed my help; it was love at first sight.

I walked toward the cart to get the pitcher of water, and she started to laugh. "Upon my ward, where did you find those jumbo pajamas?" I told her they were on my bed. Mom said better too big than too little. The nurse said she thought I must have a really smart mom. She asked me to let her roll up my sleeves and pant legs. I felt a lot better when I could see my hand and feet again.

The beginning of the end of doctors, medicine, and hospitals!

Chapter 10

I have a job!

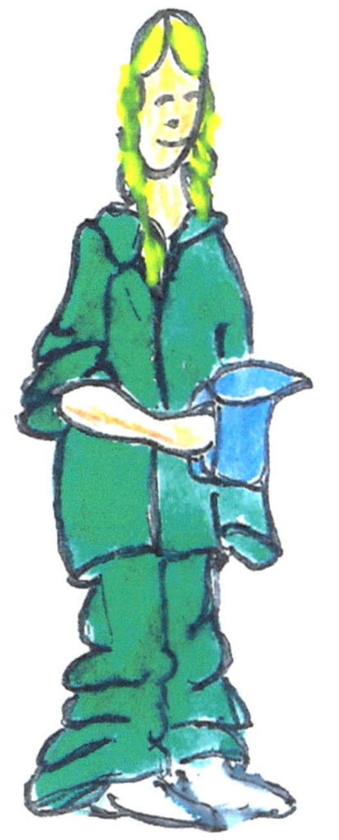

Now that I had a friend and a job, which allowed me to go all over the children's ward, I was able to meet other children who were in the hospital and other nurses who worked there and begin to feel less alone in this great big new place. The hard part about my job was that my pajamas, which were supplied by the hospital, were much bigger than I was. My new friend helped me roll up the pant leg and the sleeve, but they kept falling down. It was really hard to deliver pitchers of water when your sleeve kept falling down over the top of your hand. I was bringing water to a patient who was sitting on his bed. He noticed that I was having a problem with my sleeve. He asked me, "How come you get to deliver water?" I told him, "The nurse just asked me to help her." He was grinning at me and said, "It looks like you could use some help yourself." I asked him what he meant, and he said, "Your sleeve is in the water." I told him this was a problem; he helped me roll up my sleeves. He asked the nurse if he could help deliver water also, and she said he could. He and I finished the job of delivering water to all the beds in the children's ward.

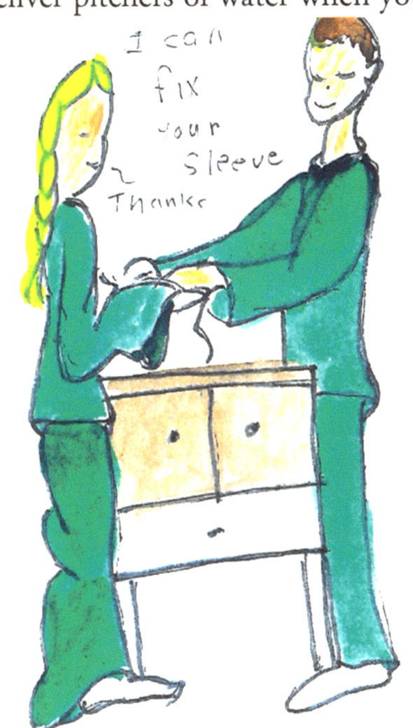

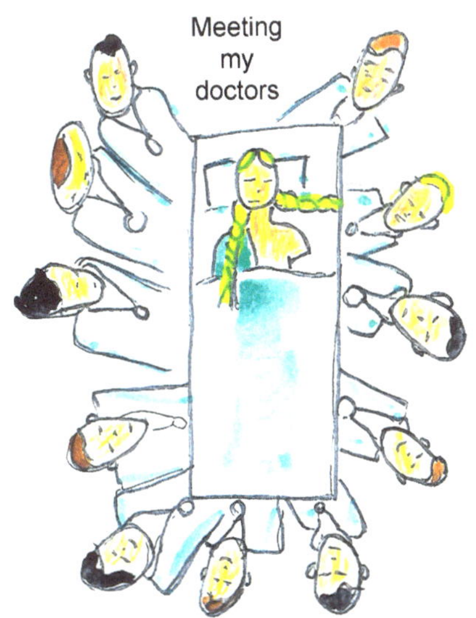
Meeting my doctors

The next day, early in the morning, before breakfast, a large number of doctors came into my cubicle and completely encircled my bed. I learned that these were student doctors who would be working with Dr. King on my case. While they were there, they looked at my arm and talked about the amputation surgery—the slow healing, which resulted in the drainage of the infection, and the surgery that would be needed to remove whatever infected parts of my arm were causing the drainage. I was very nervous and uncomfortable when I saw all these people looking at me, but after they discussed my case, Dr. King introduced all of the young doctors to me. They shook my hand, smiled, and said they were very happy to know me; and they hoped they could take care of my problem so I wouldn't have to have bandages anymore. Dr. King also told me, while they were there, that one of them would visit me every day. I felt a lot better, and I was very pleased to know that so many people were going to help me. I even felt a little bit important because I had the most doctors taking care of me of all the children in our ward.

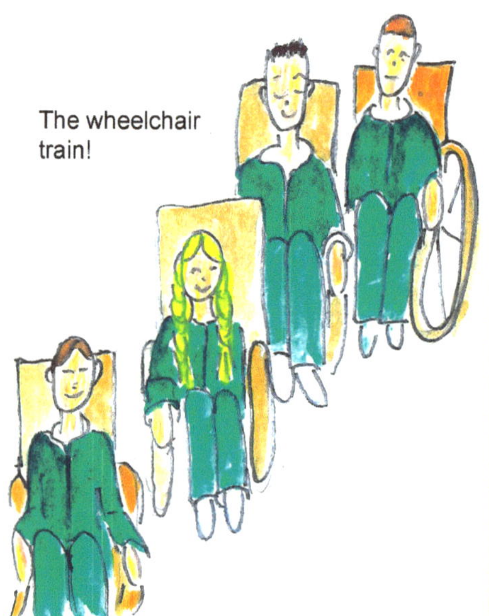
The wheelchair train!

During the day in the children's ward at Stanford-Lane Hospital, the children who could be out of bed had to move around the room in wheelchairs. The nurse told us that children were not allowed to walk around or run in the ward. I had never used a wheelchair, so I thought this would be fun. There were only four children in the ward who could move around. The other children had to stay in bed. The three other people, besides me, who could move around, were boys. They were all older and bigger than I was, and they had been using wheelchairs for longer than I had. When the nurse brought me a wheelchair, I was delighted. I thought it was going to be great fun. The nurse helped me get into the wheelchair, and then she walked away. I tried to make the wheelchair go forward. It didn't go forward; it went around in circles. I tried to push one wheel and then the other, hoping that I could make the chair go straight. It wouldn't go straight; it did go forward, but it didn't go straight. It veered one way and then the other. When I tried to push a little harder, the chair tipped over backward. I was disappointed, frustrated, and angry that it was so hard to make a wheelchair go. As I was lying on the floor after being tipped out and feeling very unhappy, the boys started laughing. Instead of crying, which I felt like doing, and being angry, I saw the humor in the situation, and I started laughing also. The boys said, "Let us help you." They had a plan. One boy would get in front of me in his wheelchair, and one would get in back. I would use the belt from my oversized robe and wrap it around the front chair so he could pull me as I held on, and the boy in back of my chair would push me. In this way, I would move forward without falling over. The third boy decided he would be the leader of the train, and we could all follow him. This idea was successful in moving me around the ward in a wheelchair. The problem was four wheelchairs careening through the children's ward, making train noises and laughter, with nurses and doctors and orderlies moving around also, a different problem needed to be reckoned with. The head nurse decided there would be no more trains in the children's ward. We could all move about in our wheelchairs. I was to try very hard and not tip over. As I was trying, in the wheelchair, to go forward, I tipped over just as one of my young doctors came to visit me. The doctor was alarmed when he saw me fall on the floor. He asked the nurse why I was in a wheelchair. She explained the rule that children could not move around unless they were in a wheelchair. The doctor asked how to change this rule. The nurse said she didn't know, but she hoped it could be changed because she was afraid that I would get hurt. My young doctor went to Dr. King and told him the situation about the wheelchair and me tipping over. Dr. King spoke with the head nurse, and it was agreed that the rules requiring that children moving around in wheelchairs would be revised. Only children who required wheelchairs to move around would use them. Children who could walk would not be required to use wheelchairs to move around in the ward. That was the best news we could have received. There were a lot of children we wanted to visit—the ones who couldn't leave their beds. The wheelchairs were too large to visit in the cubicles, but without chairs, we could walk in and talk to children who couldn't get out of bed. We could play checkers or cards, play with paper dolls, read or tell stories to one another to make a long day go faster.

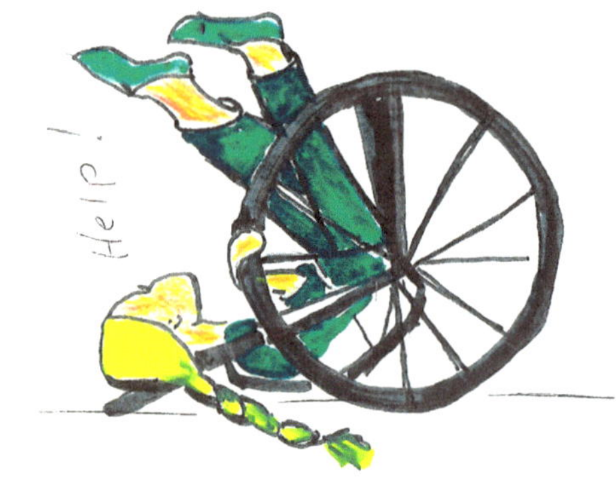

Some of the really special people we had in our ward were the candy stripers and student nurses. They came every day and read stories to us, played games with us, and sometimes just sat and held a child who was sad, lonely, or frightened. They were always young and pretty, and all of us loved them.

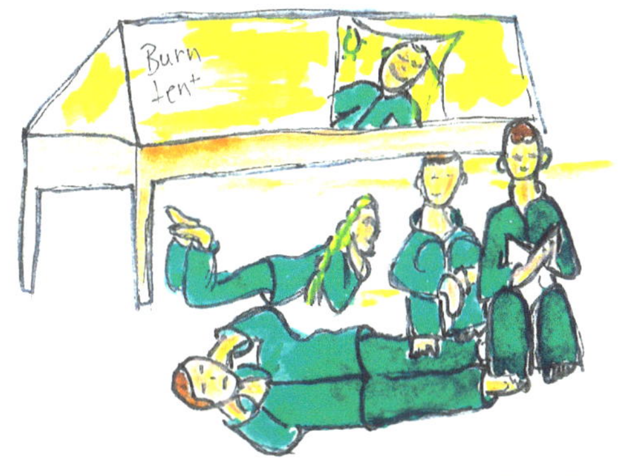

One of the children we all wanted to know was the boy who had been burned. His burns covered so much of his body that he was isolated to protect him from getting infections. The whole front part of his body had been burned during an accident when he inadvertently caused a tub of boiling water to spill down the front of him. He had been in the hospital for a long time before I came. His cubicle was next to mine. He couldn't have blankets or sheets or anything touch his skin. He had a tent over his body with a light in it to keep him warm. I think he was ten years old, and he was getting better. At night, after the lights were turned off in the ward, the boys who could get out of bed and I would go visit him. We couldn't walk around the ward after the lights were off, but the glass wall in our cubicles were open about two feet above the floor so we could crawl under the cubicle walls to visit him. One of the boys who had been part of the "train" was a very good reader. He would bring storybooks and read to all of us deep into the night by the light of the tent that kept the boy with the burns warm. Sometimes we just talked about what had happened to us and why we were at Stanford-Lane Hospital. We learned that all of us were there because we had very special medical cases.

Most of us had had life-threatening experiences. It was a wonderful thing to know that you are not the only person that everybody thought was going to die. We felt a very special relationship for one another because we were survivors; we were getting better, and all of us knew we were going to be just fine. We also felt that we were special because Stanford-Lane Hospital only accepted very special cases to their teaching hospital, and therefore, all of us must be very special children.

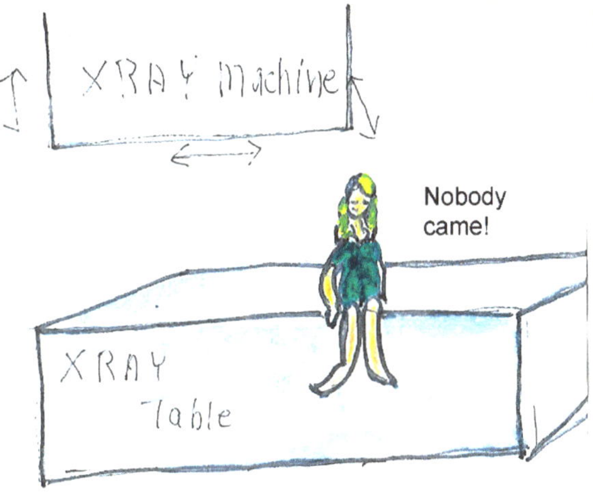

The beginning of the second week that I was at the hospital in San Francisco, everything changed. I no longer had time to play with my friends. I spent a lot of time being x-rayed in the biggest x-ray room I had ever seen. They wanted to take x-rays of the stump of my arm from every angle. To do this, they put me on a large metal table that could tilt up or down and sideways. The camera was as big as a bus and would come down very close to my arm. I was terrified. The metal table was ice cold; the room was cold too. I was freezing, and I needed to go to the bathroom. I told the nurse, and she said it would only be a little while, and then I could get down and go. After she told me this, she left. There was no one in the room with me. The metal table was probably four feet off the floor I couldn't get off it. I waited. I was getting desperate. I called. Nobody came. I called as loud as I could. I sat up on the table and yelled for somebody to please come and help me. Nobody came. I couldn't hear anybody. I wondered if they had forgotten me. I started to cry; I cried very hard and kept yelling for somebody to come. Nobody came. I wet my pants, and I cried and cried and cried. When the nurse came in to the x-ray room, she asked why I was crying. I explained to her that I had called and called, and nobody came. I needed to go the bathroom. "You told me it would just be a little while. But it was a long time, and I am very embarrassed, and I want to go home because I don't like this place anymore." She put her arms around me and held me close while I cried. She said she was very sorry; she had taken the film someplace; it took longer than she expected. She told me she would give me a shower and nice clean pajamas before I went back to the ward. I stopped crying. I dried my eyes and said, "You know I am not a baby. I don't have accidents like this, but I forgive you."

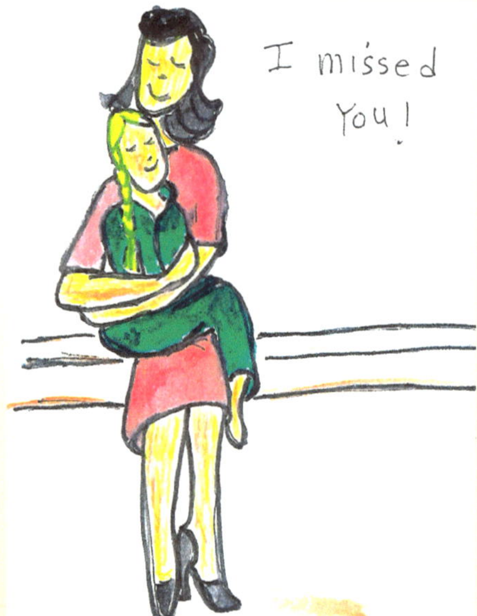

After the x-rays were done, there were a lot of tests. Some required taking blood, measuring my arm and the stump of my arm, and many other tests. There were new medicines that I was taking. I don't know what they were for, but they made me feel sick.

My mother came to visit me the day before my surgery. I was so happy to see her. She held me in her arms; we kissed and hugged. She told me about my little brother, Donnie. He was really cute and funny and asked for me. She told me about Tyke going to school and that she missed me and that everybody wanted me to get better and come home. She told me she came to San Francisco on the train. Grandma Souza, her mother, had met the train in Sacramento; and my sister, Tyke, and my little brother, Donnie, stayed in Sacramento with her while Mom visited me at the hospital.

Early the next morning, Mom was in my cubicle holding my hand as she assured me the surgery would soon be over, and I would be able to get well. One of my young doctors and a nurse came into my cubicle and put me on the gurney. Mom stayed in my cubicle as I was wheeled out of the cubicle through the ward, out the door into the hall, and down to surgery.

This is the day I had been waiting for. Hopefully, this surgery was going to take care of all the problems keeping me from getting well. If they could stop the drainage in my arm, it would heal. When it was healed, I wouldn't have to change the bandages every day. If I didn't have to change the bandages every day, I wouldn't have tape burn on my arm and shoulder, and it would not hurt. If everything went well, I wouldn't have to go to the doctor every day, so I could go to school.

Happy day!

Chapter II

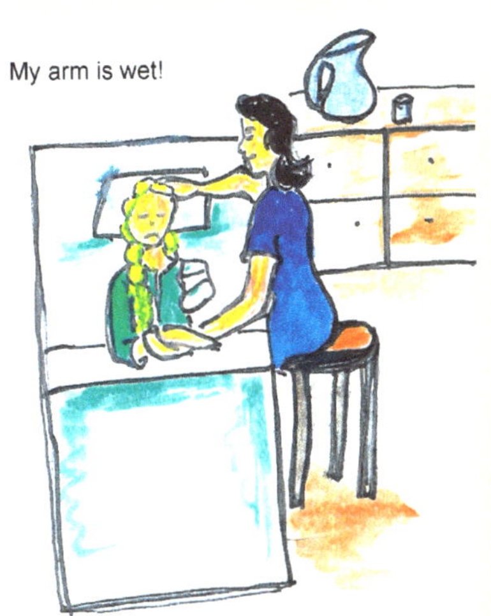

The next thing I remember, I was back in my cubicle; it was nighttime. It was dark except for a small light in the cubicle. My mother was sitting by my bed. She looked worried, and she was holding my hand. I felt terrible, my head hurt, I ached all over, and the stump of my arm felt wet. I asked my mother what had happened. She said the surgery was over, and the doctors thought I would soon be getting well. I told her I needed a towel. She asked me why. I told her because the stump of my arm felt wet. She said it wasn't wet. It was wrapped in bandages, and the bandages were dry. I told her I wanted to look at it and see why it felt wet. She told me the doctors didn't want me moving around. I tried to sit up so I could see why that area felt so strange. When I lifted my head to look at my arm, I felt very sick and had to lie down. Mom said I should wait and talk to the doctors tomorrow when they come to see me. I told her I was very thirsty, and she gave me some ice to suck on. She said that drinking water after surgery could make me sick. I don't know how long my mother stayed with me that night, or if she stayed all night. The next morning, when I woke up, she was there sitting in the same place, still holding my hand.

The nurse came in to my cubicle and told my mother she should go eat breakfast while the doctors checked to see how I was doing. Mom said she would rather stay and talk to the doctors when they came in to see me. The nurse said the doctors wanted to talk to her also, but they would have a conference around my bed to see how my recovery was going before they talked to her. Mom went to have breakfast. The nurse washed my face, straightened my bed, recorded my temperature and blood pressure, and asked how I felt and if I wanted something to eat. I told her I didn't feel good. I didn't want to eat.

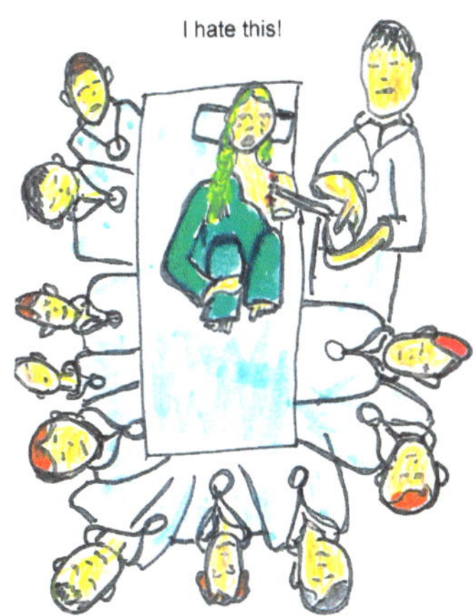

The doctors came in and stood around my bed. They asked me how I felt. I told them I felt awful, but I was most worried because my arm was wet and sticky. I told them I wanted to know what they had done and why it felt wet. The doctors helped me sit up in bed. Then they took the bandages off the stump of my arm. I couldn't believe what I saw. There was a tube coming out of the side of the stump of my arm, and it was held in place with wire. Wrapped all around the bottom of the stump of my arm was a rubber sheet that was held in place with tape. The drainage from the unhealed area near the bone was now coming out of the side of my arm instead of the bottom that's why it felt wet.

The bandages absorbed the drainage, but the rubber sheet stayed wet. I asked why they did that. That wet sheet felt terrible, and I hated it. It was cold and wet, and I didn't want it on me. The tube was ugly, and the wire hurt. I didn't want wires in my arm. The doctors explained that the area that was causing the drainage was in my shoulder. They had to remove my shoulder cap and scrape all of the infected area clean. The bottom of the stump of my arm was then stitched closed so that it would no longer drain. They also explained why they wanted the rubber sheet instead of bandages. They wanted to extract the fluid and analyze it daily to see if it was free of bacteria. Then they showed me a little bulblike structure also made of rubber that could be squeezed at the end of the tube that was wired into my arm to draw out the fluid. I asked if I needed a shoulder cap. The doctor said I could live without one. He said they didn't want to take it out, but the infection had settled deep in the bones of the shoulder cap, and there was no way they could save that and still have me get well.

The doctor said, "I'm going to show you how this will be done." He put the little bulb on the end of the tube that was wired into the side of my arm and began to squeeze it. I screamed! I will never forget how badly that hurt. It felt like a broken tooth with ice in it. He stopped squeezing and asked me what was wrong. I told him it felt like a toothache all over my body. The doctor said, "This operation has to be done three times a day until the drainage stops." I told him I didn't think I could do it three times a day. The doctors discussed the various options and decided they would give me a shot of Novocain before each procedure to help with the pain. Then they gave me a shot of Novocain, waited a few minutes, and squeezed the bulb again. It was terribly painful. I gritted my teeth and clenched my fist until the squeezing stopped. I had tears, but I did not cry. If it had to be done, I could do it.

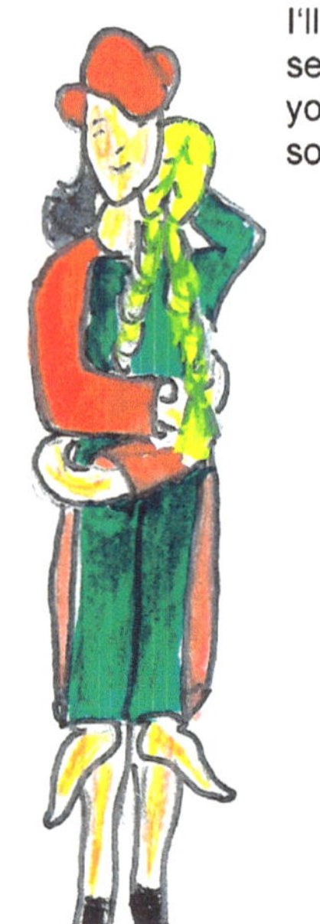

When my mother returned from breakfast, she met with the doctors. They explained what had happened and how I had reacted and felt. Then they brought her into the cubicle and showed her the wired in tube on the side of the stump of my arm. They told her that they had removed my shoulder cap and why it had to be done. My mother began to cry just before she left the cubicle.

Later, my mother came in to see me and told me she was going to stay for another day. I knew she had planned to go home the day after the surgery. So I knew she was worried about the wired in tube. I was glad she was going to stay, but I was sorry she was sad.

When my mother came to see me the next day, I was feeling a little better. I couldn't get out of bed. I couldn't even move around very much because I was sore. Mom spent most of the day with me, and then she had to go catch the train. She said she hated to go, but I told her I was fine. We hugged, and she kissed me good-bye and promised to be back in a week.

I'm not sure how many days they had to drain the fluid from my wound. But even with the Novocain, it was very painful. I felt unwell most of the time and dreaded the next procedure before the present one was finished. The nurses and the candy stripers and some of my friends in the ward came by to visit me, but I just didn't feel good enough to visit.

Soon I was feeling better. The draining procedure was over. The wire had been taken out of my shoulder. Things were healing, and I knew I was better. I could enjoy the stories by the light of the burn patient's tent. Most of my playmates, the ones who were mobile, had had surgeries and were sick or had gone home. It was lonely without them. The boy with the burns and I talked a lot. He said he would miss me when I went home. He said he could tell I would be going home soon because I was almost well. I knew he was right. I was a lot better. I was glad I was better. I liked him a lot, and I told him I would miss him too.

A few days later, my mom came in to the ward with my favorite young doctor, the one who took care of me most of the time. They were smiling and looking very happy. Mom took my hand and said, "Today is the day you go home." I kissed her. I hugged her, and I said, "Do you mean it?" Mom said, "I can take you home just as soon as the doctor checks you over and we get the paperwork.

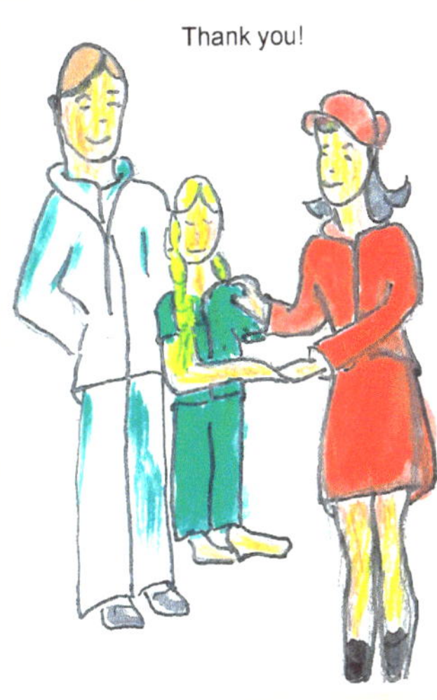

The young doctor, I can't remember his name, had seen me almost every day that I was in the hospital at Stanford-Lane. I felt that he was one of my best friends because when things got bad, he was there to make me feel better. He always answered my questions, and he told me the truth. He was a lot like Dr. McKnight but much younger.

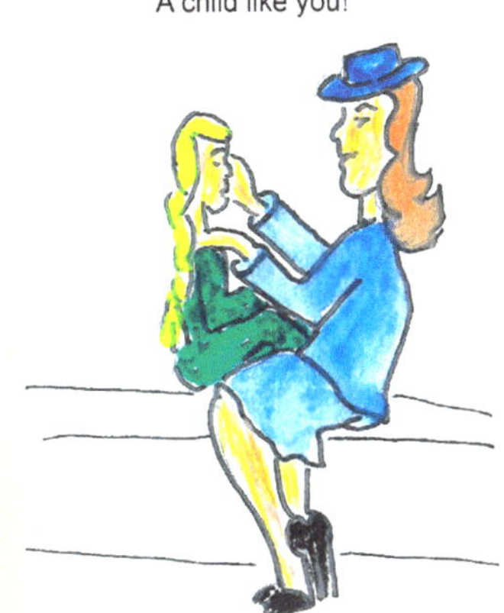

That day, he told me his wife was coming to visit me because he had talked about me so much that she wanted to meet me. She came to the children's ward just before Mom came to take me home. We sat on my bed in my cubicle; and she told me that of all the children her husband had worked with, he thought I was the strongest, the toughest, and the bravest child he had ever known. She told me she was going to have a baby soon, and she and her husband hoped that their child would be like me.

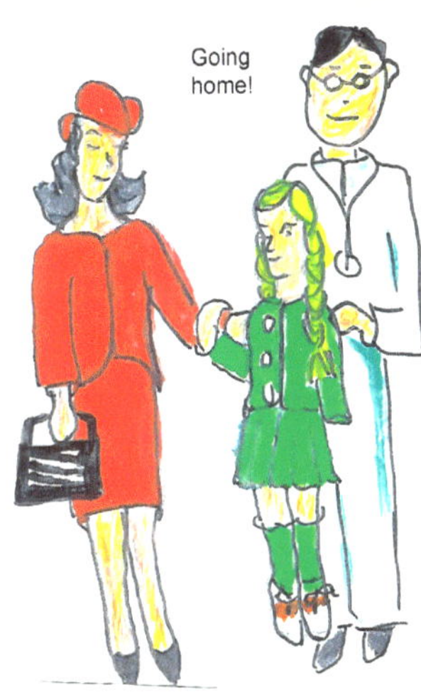

When Mom came back to take me home, Dr. King was with her. He said he came to say good-bye and wish me luck. I hugged him and thanked him for all his help. I hugged the young doctor and his wife and thanked them for all they had done. Mom shook their hands and thanked everybody. As we walked to the door on our way out of the children's ward, my dear friend, the nurse who let me help her give the children water, came to say good-bye. We hugged and kissed, and then Mom took my hand, and we left Stanford-Lane children's ward

We were on our way home!

Chapter 12

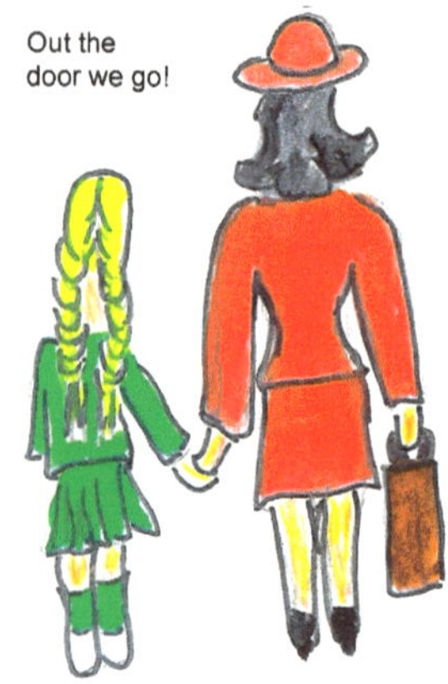

With my hand in one of Mom's hands and a suitcase in her other, we walked out of the children's ward, into the hall to the elevator, down several floors to a large receiving room. This room was bright with sunshine and noisy with people. Across the room were two huge doors leading to the street. We walked out of the hospital down the sidewalk to the streetcar stop. Mom asked how I felt. I told her I felt wonderful. She said we could either take the streetcar or a cab to the ferry building. I said okay. I didn't care how we got home. I just wanted to go. She asked me if I thought I could get on the streetcar by myself. I said, "Of course I can get on the streetcar by myself." She asked if I felt tired or weak. I said, "No, I am fine. Let's go!"

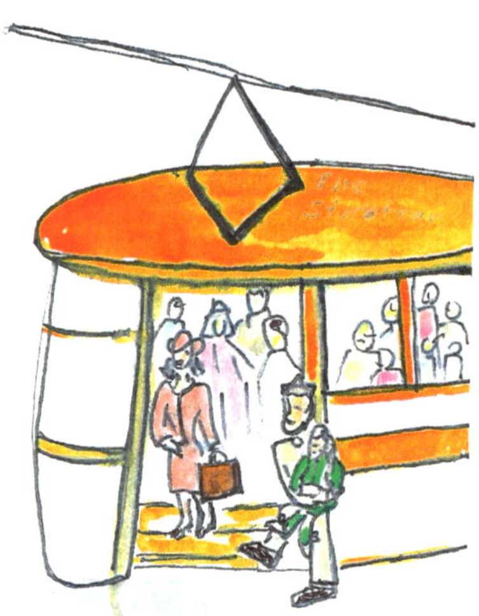

The streetcar stopped right in front of us. It was very full. Mom walked up the steps, put down her suitcase, and turned around to help me up the steps. When she turned around, she saw that a tall young soldier had picked me up and put me on the streetcar. Mom thanked him for helping me, and I thanked him too. The soldier asked us where we were going. We told him we were going to the ferry then cross the bay and take the train to Sacramento where my brother and sister would join us, and we would all go home to Portola. He said he had just left the hospital. He had been wounded in a battle in the Pacific. He was going home. He had not seen his family in two years. I told him I had just come out of the hospital too. He asked me what had happened to me. I told him I had fallen and broken my arm, and it had been infected with gangrene, and the doctor had to cut it off, and penicillin saved my life. He looked sad; I think he was crying. He turned away from us. I looked at Mom; she looked sad too. I didn't know what to say, so I didn't say anything. I just looked at all the people on the sidewalk as the streetcar traveled toward the ferry building.

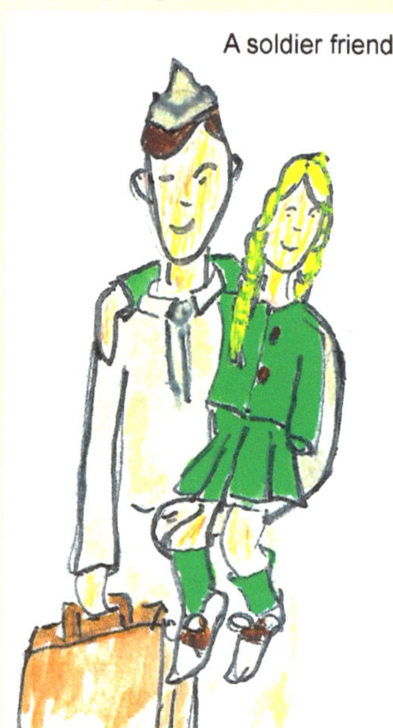

When we got by the ferry building, the streetcar traveled on a track that turned like a half circle that stopped right in front of several very large doors leading into the building. The soldier took Mom's suitcase in one hand and lifted me up with his other to help us off the streetcar. We thanked him again and walked into the ferry building. The building was big and very interesting. There were lots of people. There were little open shops where you could buy things to eat, to wear, and toys to play with. Mom and I bought toys for Donnie and Tyke, my baby brother and my little sister, who were staying with Grandma in Sacramento. Mom and I had a cup of hot cocoa while we waited for the ferry.

When the ferry came, we had to walk up a broad wooden slanting walkway right onto the ship. There were lots of people, and Mom held on to my hand very tightly so I wouldn't get lost. She also was carrying a suitcase. Then a sailor asked if he could carry the suitcase for her. She said thank you and asked him where he had been. He said he'd seen action in the Pacific and had been wounded and was on his way home.

He asked about what had happened to me. I didn't want to make him sad, so I didn't say anything. Mom told him what happened to me, and he said he was very sorry that I had been so sick, but he was glad I was better and going home.

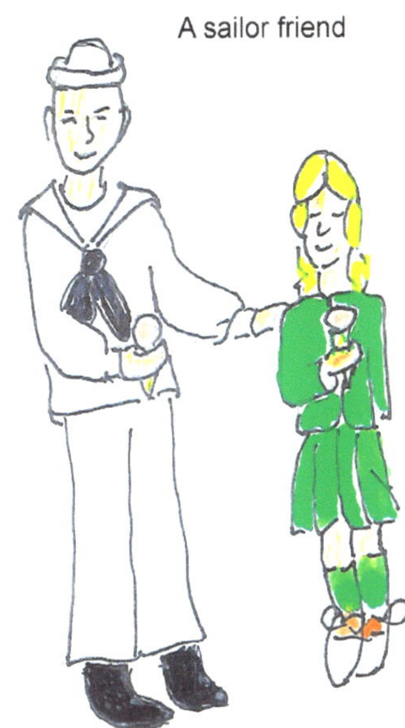
A sailor friend

When we got on the ferry, we went upstairs to stand on the deck and watch San Francisco move away as we headed for Oakland where the train was waiting for us. It was the ferry that was really moving; it just seemed like San Francisco was moving away as we watched. It felt so good to be outside—to smell the ocean, feel the wind in my hair, and watch the birds fly all around the ship. Most of the people on the ferry were military. Most of them had been wounded and were going home. We talked to many soldiers and sailors that day on the ferry and then later on the train. It seemed like every soldier on the train came to talk to me and my mom. They took turns carrying me back and forth on the train. They said there were soldiers and sailors they wanted me to meet, and they took me from car to car on the train and introduced me to other people. They said we were all veterans of different wars. Some of the soldiers had children who were eight years old, and they hadn't seen them for four years. One soldier told me that his son was about my age now. The last time he had seen him he was about four. They sang songs to me and bought me soda pop and ice cream. I had a great time playing with the soldiers and sailors.

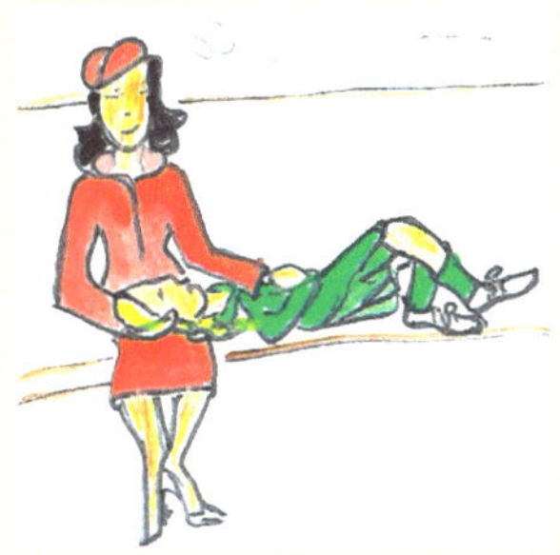

After a while, Mom told the soldiers that I needed to rest. I told Mom I was having fun, and I wasn't a bit tired. She explained that I had had surgery only the week before. The soldiers very gently sat me down next to Mom and thanked me. I thanked them for a very good time. I didn't know what they thanked me for. I fell asleep within minutes after the soldiers left. I slept all the way to Sacramento. Mom woke me as we came in to the station.

How is Yvonne?
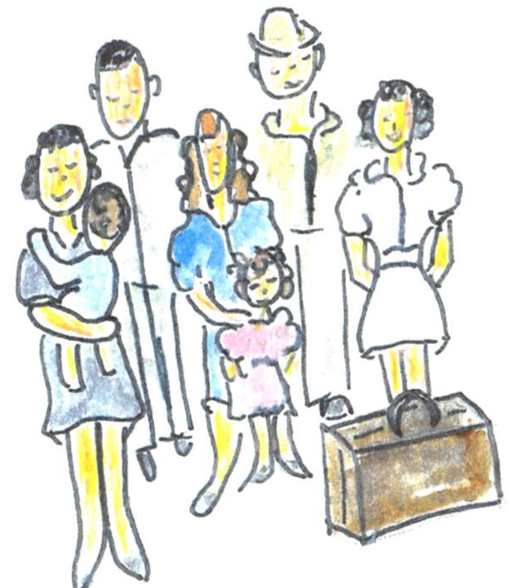

When the train stopped in Sacramento, my grandma Sousa, my uncle Joe, my uncle Alfred and aunt Jesse, my godmother Teeny, and Tyke and Donnie were all there to meet the train. Mom and I did not get off the train. All the family was there to see Mom and me and to bring my brother and sister to the train so we could all go home together. Everyone wanted to see how I was and ask Mom if I was through with doctors and hospitals. Mom told them I was better, but I would have to go back for a checkup in June. Uncle Joe helped Tyke get on the train, and Grandma handed Donnie to my mother. Uncle Alfred put the suitcases and toys that

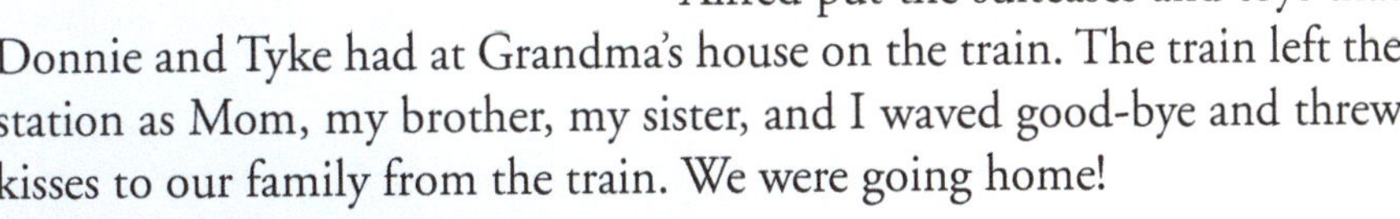
Donnie and Tyke had at Grandma's house on the train. The train left the station as Mom, my brother, my sister, and I waved good-bye and threw kisses to our family from the train. We were going home!

Good-bye!
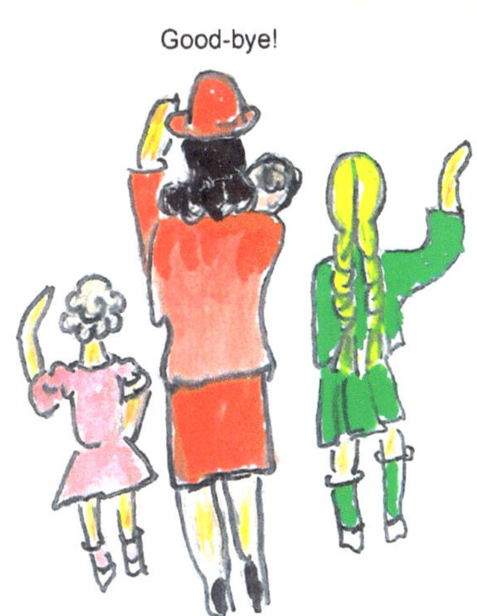

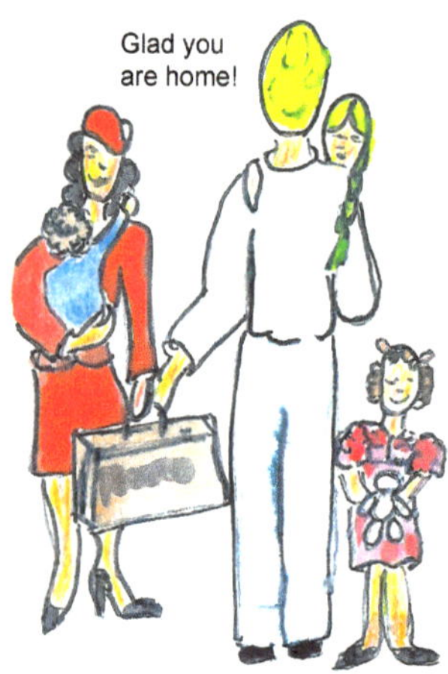

About seven hours later, the train finally pulled into Portola station. Dad was waiting for us. When we got off the train, Mom let me go first. Daddy lifted me off the train. Dad held me in his arms. He held me very tightly; then he looked at me and said, "Are you really okay?" I said, "Yes, I feel great." Then he said he was so glad we were all home. Tyke got off the train and stood by Daddy. Mom and Donnie got off the train and handed a suitcase to Daddy.

Our family was all together again.

Chapter 13

Portola in 1943 was a very small town. Its major and most important industry was the Western Pacific Railroad. The town population had grown with the fierceness and intensity of World War II. My father was one of the many railroad men who were transferred to Portola because of the war effort. Housing the families of these workers was a major problem. This little town had one hotel, a few small homes, a grocery store, a drugstore, a small department store, a school, and a few churches. Building new homes was a low priority because acquiring building materials was nearly impossible.

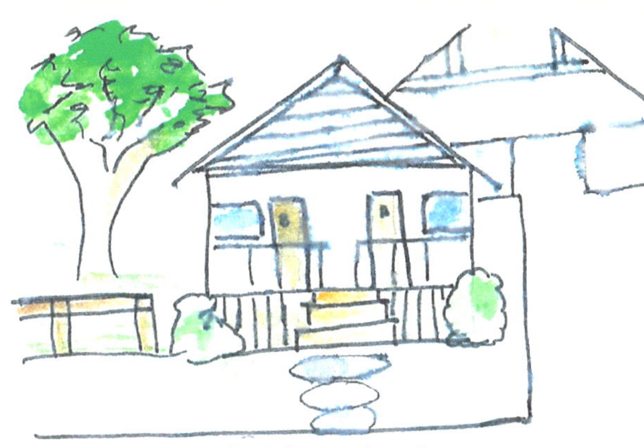

Portola apartment

We lived in an apartment. We had the largest apartment in the building because we were the largest family. Our apartment had one large bedroom, a rather small living room, and a very large kitchen. Our apartment also shared a large front porch with all the other people who lived there. The window in the living room of our apartment faced onto the porch. The bedroom had two windows—one faced the street, the other faced the driveway that ran the length of the house to a barn at the back. Behind the kitchen was a small back porch. The large bedroom had two double beds and chests of drawers for clothes. My parents slept in one bed, and my sister and I slept in the other one.

Midnight snack

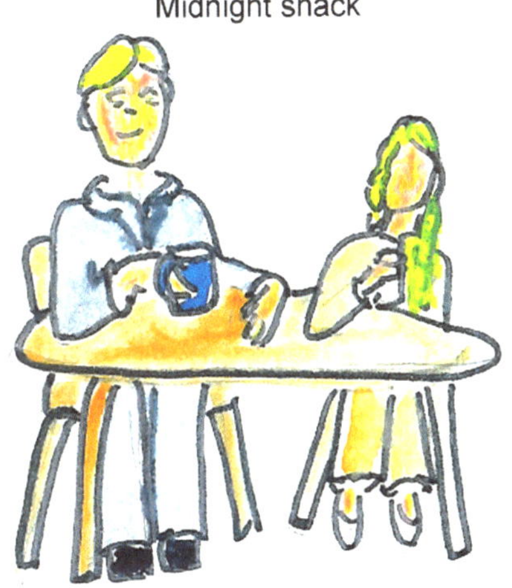

After I got hurt, I had trouble sleeping in a bed with anyone else. I was a restless sleeper. I had nightmares that would cause me to wake up screaming or crying in the middle of the night. My parents asked the doctor what caused the nightmares I was having. He said he wasn't sure, but because many of the nightmares were about falling, he thought perhaps going from the tall hospital bed to the lower regular bed may have caused a problem for me. He suggested that I sleep by myself in my own bed instead of sleeping with my sister. My parents put a small twin bed in the kitchen right under the window. I liked sleeping in there because if anybody was up and about, they would be in the kitchen. I liked to visit with my father when he came home from work at midnight. We often had a midnight snack together. I also liked to be awake when Mom got up to make breakfast in the morning. Sometimes she would let me help. It was nice for Mom and me to have a quiet time together. Another reason I moved into the kitchen to sleep was that the baby needed a bed close to my parents. All in all it was a pretty comfortable arrangement.

I was home because the surgery had been successful. However, I was still wearing bandages over the wound in my arm. I thought when I came home from the hospital, this time I would be well, not just better.

The day after we got home from San Francisco, the whole family was having breakfast in the kitchen. Everybody was happy and talking about our trip home, about the fun that Tyke had at Grandma's house, how much Donnie had grown while I had been in the hospital. Daddy was so happy to have us home. Being home was very special to all of us. I wanted to know when I was going to go to school.

Mom looked at Dad, and they both looked at me. Mom said, "Tomorrow we will see Dr. McKnight, who will give you a complete checkup and let us know if you're ready to go to school." That answer did not make me happy. I thought that I could go to school as soon as I got home. I had the surgery; the doctors and everybody said that it had been a success. I felt just fine. I wanted to go to school. I didn't want to have to go to the doctor. I was better. It wasn't fair. I was tired of being sick. I didn't want to be sick anymore. I wanted to be like everybody else. I wanted to go to school. I started crying. As I tried to get out of the chair, it fell over. My father yelled at me. He said, "Young lady, you will go to school just as soon as the doctors say you can." I threw myself on the bed and cried.

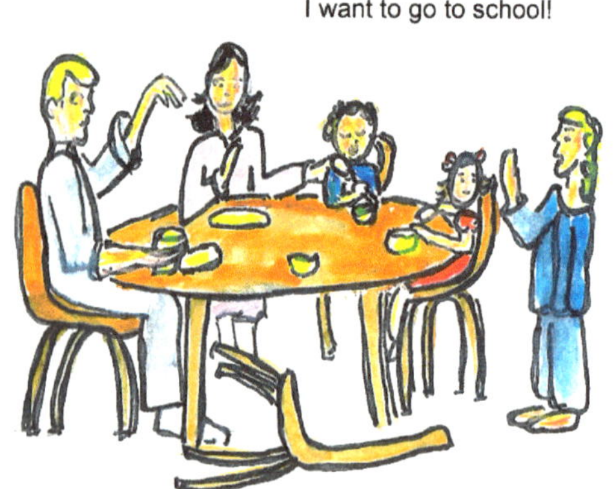

The next morning, we had breakfast as usual. My sister was dressed for school. When she left to go to school, she said, "Don't worry, you'll get to go to school soon." My mother put clothes out for me to wear to visit the doctor at his office at the hospital. I dressed myself while Mom dressed the baby and herself. My aunt came and drove us to the hospital for my appointment. I was very sad and unhappy. I thought as soon as the surgery was over and I came home from San Francisco, I would be all better. If I was all better, then I could go to school, play with other kids, and be like everybody else.

When Dr. McKnight found out we were there to see him, he came in to his office with a big smile on his face and said, "How are you? I am so happy to see you! You look great. How did things go in San Francisco? Did you like Dr. King? Are you glad to be home?" I didn't say anything. My mother was holding the baby, and she didn't say anything either. Dr. McKnight asked, "Is something wrong?" Mom looked at me and told the doctor that I wasn't happy. Then Dr. McKnight looked at me. I told him that I was disappointed that I couldn't go to school this morning with my sister. He told me he wanted to see how my vital signs were, how my wound looked from the surgery, how tall I was, and how much I weighed. He said he hoped I could go to school next week. I wanted to know why I had to wait. I had the surgery, and everybody said I was fine, and I could come home from San Francisco, so I thought I was all better. Why did I have to wait another week? Dr. McKnight took my hand and brought me close to him. He said, "You are better, but you have been very sick. I want you to go to school, and your mom and dad want you to go to school, and everybody in this town wants you to go to school. But when you have been as sick as you were, it takes awhile to get well. You are so much better than you were. Remember when you lay in bed all day, and you couldn't walk, you felt bad most of the time, you couldn't go home or play with other children?" I said, "Yes, I remember, but I didn't know I would have to wait after I got home from San Francisco. I thought I was all better. Everybody said the surgery in San Francisco would make me all better."

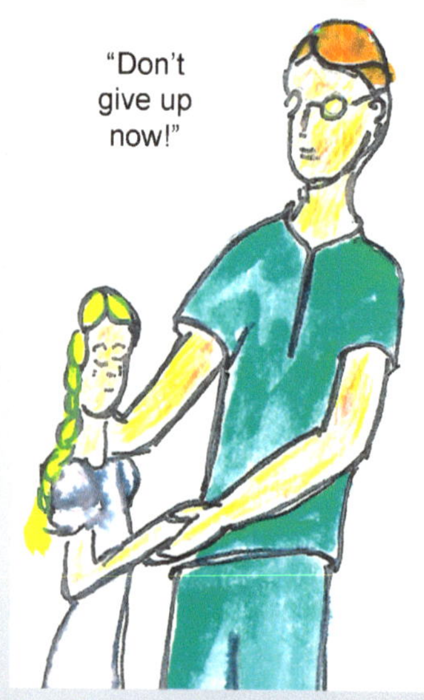

Dr. McKnight examined my arm, checked my blood pressure and my temperature. He measured my height, weighed me, and asked me to walk around the room so we could check my posture. Then he sat down and told me that my blood pressure, my temperature, my weight and height, and posture were good. The wound in my arm was healing and looked good. He worried that I might fall or bump my arm in some way at school that could open the stitches. It was decided that I would wait another week and check everything again, hopefully take the stitches out, and then I should be able to go to school. I looked at him as tears were leaking out of my eyes. I told him I didn't think I would ever be well. He said, "I know it has been a long time, and you have been very brave. Don't give up now." Mom gave me a hanky. I wiped the tears away. I said, "Okay, if I have to wait, I will."

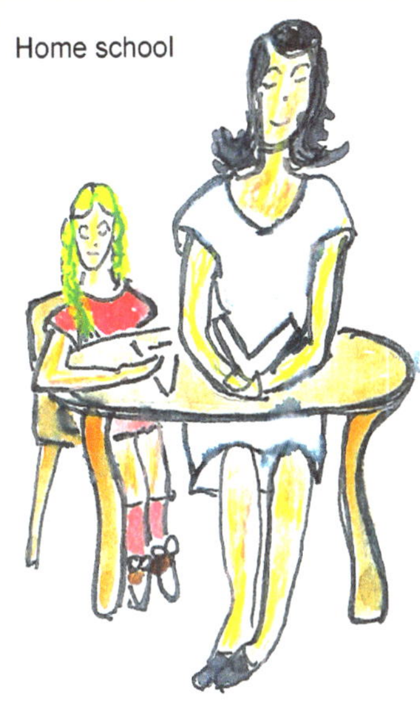
Home school

On the way home from the doctor's office, we stopped at the library, and Mom and I selected some books. Some were for her to read to me, and some were for me to read to her. I decided if I had to wait another week, I should probably start practicing my reading. I told Mom that I need to practice arithmetic also. Our next stop was at the dime store where we got some tablets for writing both numbers and letters. I had plenty of color crayons at home.

Every day after my sister went to school, Mom and I played school. First I would read to her, and that was hard because I didn't know very many words. The reading class lasted thirty minutes. Then we stopped. I took a break and played with the baby and had a snack. I would lie on my little bed, and Mom would read a story. I usually fell asleep because trying to read wore me out. After my nap, we had thirty minutes of arithmetic. This was fun because we used playing cards and played Fish, which is a great game for young children to learn about numbers. After arithmetic, we took another break. We played with the baby and had another snack. Then we would lie on my bed in the kitchen, and Mom would read me another story. Donnie and I, and sometimes Mom, would fall asleep during our story.

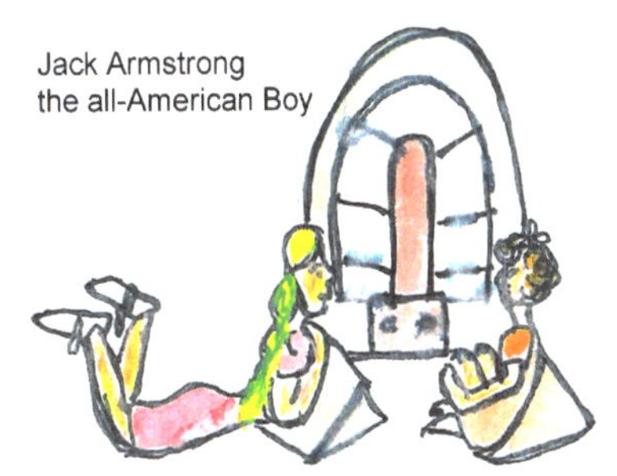
Jack Armstrong the all-American Boy

An hour of school was exhausting for me. After our morning school lesson, I often slept all afternoon. When Tyke got home from school, I would ask her what she did, and she would share with me and tell me about her friends and her teacher. She would show me her homework, her reading book, and whatever pictures and things she had from school. Then I would tell her about school with Mom and Donnie. I would show her the book I was reading and the numbers and pictures I had made at home. Then she read her story from school to me, and I would read the story that I had practiced that morning with Mom. It was fun to feel normal, doing normal things that other kids were doing. After we shared our schoolwork, we would listen to the radio. *Captain Midnight* and *Jack Armstrong, the All-American Boy* were two of our favorite shows.

The next week, we went to see Dr. McKnight as planned. He was waiting for us and, as usual, seemed very happy to see us. He asked me how my week had been and what I had been doing since I'd seen him last. I told him about going to the library and the dime store. I told about having homeschool with Mom, and I told him about sharing my sister's school lessons and my homeschool lessons in the afternoon when she came home from school. He clapped his hands with great delight. "I am so proud of you," he said. "That was exactly the right thing to do to get ready to go back to school. So let's see how you look today."

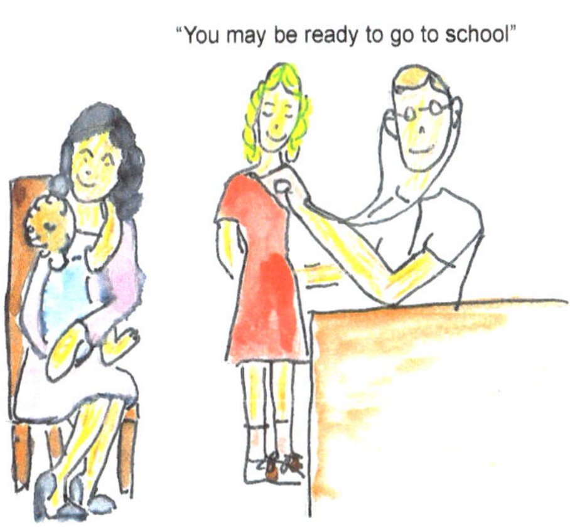
"You may be ready to go to school"

After the examination, he told me everything looked good. He took the stitches out of my arm and covered the wound with a Band-Aid. It was a big Band-Aid but much smaller and lighter and cooler than the bandages I had needed.

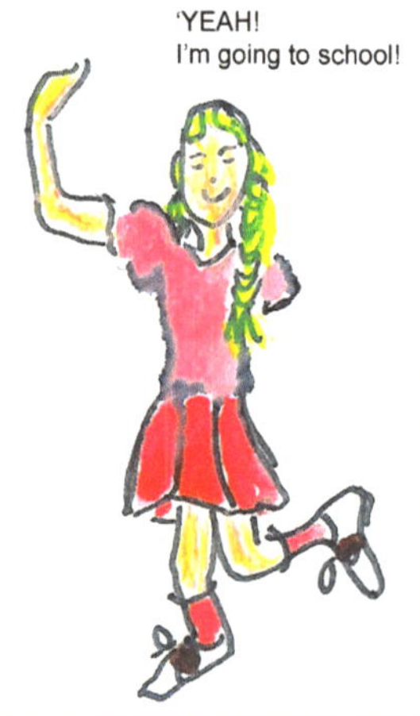

The doctor sat down next to me and said, "It's time to talk about going to school." I said, "I am ready!" The doctor affirmed, "I see that you are, and you have planned for it. I think you could start school next week. It's now the first of April, and school will be over in June for this year. You are making excellent progress, but you only have two full months left of school. I think you and your parents should go to the school and talk about a special schedule for you. Homeschooling has been an hour long in the morning. I think going to school for an hour in the morning with two breaks would be perfect for you. I think if you try to do more than that, it will be too much, and you would be very disappointed if you had to drop out. On the other hand, if you find that you're not tired after the morning session, and the teachers agree, I see no reason why we can't add time and activities to your schedule."

"Okay, I can begin school on Monday. I can go to school for one hour in the morning. But if I feel better, I can go longer. That's a deal!"

My mother and I would go to the school and talk to the principal. I would take a reading class and an arithmetic class.

"I'm going to school on Monday. Yeah!"

Chapter 14

After we met with Dr. McKnight, I continued homeschooling for the rest of the week. We kept our routine of one-half hour of reading and language arts and one-half hour of numbers and arithmetic. By the end of the week, I was feeling very confident about being able to go to school.

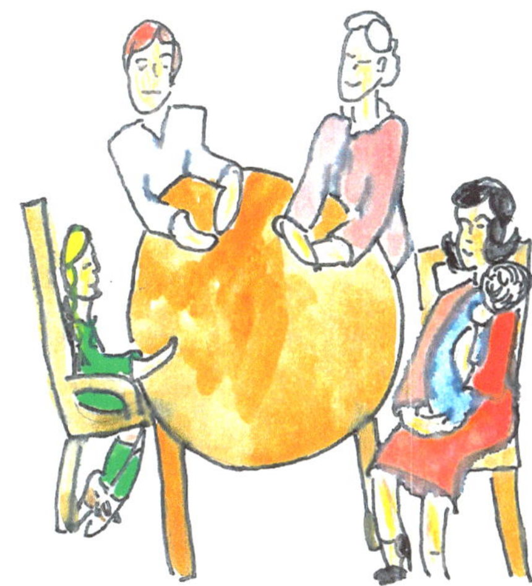

Mom made an appointment to meet with the principal and a second grade teacher at the Portola Elementary School. Mom and I introduced ourselves. They told us their names and asked us to sit with them at a table in the principal's office. Mom asked me to tell the ladies why we had asked for this meeting. I stood up and looked at the principal and said, "I want to go to school more than anything in the world." Mrs. Palmer, the teacher, smiled at me and said, "A wise claim for one so young." Mom told them that I had hurt my arm in August of 1943. It was now April of 1944. I had been in the hospital in Portola and in San Francisco much of that time. The only schooling I had had in that time was two weeks of homeschooling that began when I returned from the hospital in San Francisco two weeks ago and included a half hour of reading and language arts and a half hour of numbers and arithmetic. My mother explained to them that I was getting better but that I was still weak, underweight, and in the process of healing. We were very hopeful that they could develop a schedule that would allow me to come to school.

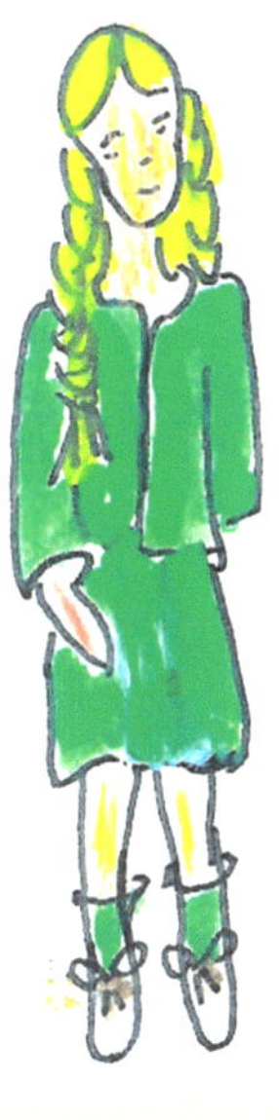

The principal asked if we understood that there were only two months of school left, and with my health issues and special needs, it would be difficult to put a program together.

My mother told them that we understood we were asking a lot from them in order to meet my needs. She tried to explain to them how important it was for me to go to school, be in a class, and do the normal things done by children.

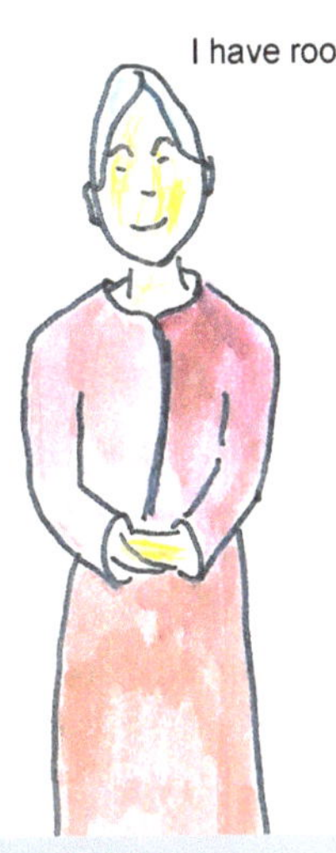

The second grade teacher was a very old lady and had taught school for a long time. She smiled, and I thought she was beautiful. She said, "Of course the principal is certainly correct about the days left. It's very late in the school year, but we do have a special class in language arts and a special class in numbers. It just so happens that both of these classes are one-half hour long. I believe the language arts class starts at 9:30. After that class, there is a short recess, and the number class begins at 10:10 and lasts until 10:40. After the number class, the children from the special classes join the regular class for recess and classes in music, PE, or art. Each day of the week, the regular class offers one of these electives for all the children in both the special and regular classes."

The principal said, "The special classes could be a possibility. I don't think you can get caught up to grade level in two half-hour classes a day. Do you understand that you will be in second grade again next year even if you can come to school these two months?

If there is a second grade teacher who would be willing to do the extra planning to meet your need and you understand that you will have to repeat second grade." She was looking at me. "I support the idea."

"Mom, did you hear that? I get to go to Portola Elementary School." Mom asked, "Is there a teacher who would do that for Yvonne?"

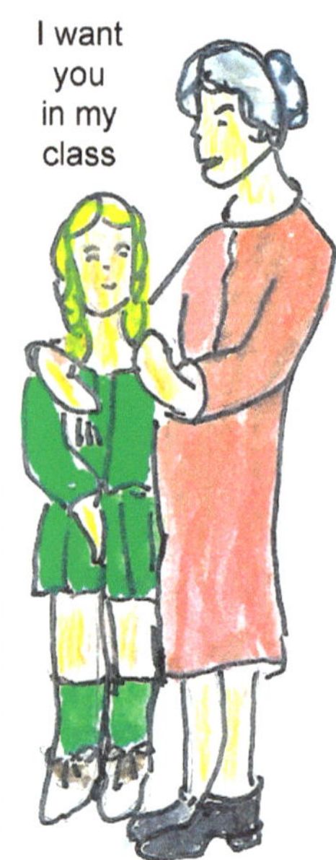

The principal said she would have to investigate and see if there was a teacher who would take another student and would be willing to do the extra work. Mrs. Palmer was the name of the second grade teacher at our meeting. She said she had room in her class, and she would love the opportunity to work with me.

The principal said, "If you are willing to do this extra work, Mrs. Palmer, begin with the one-hour program. If it appears after the first week Yvonne is well enough to add another half hour, we will meet with her mother and make the adjustment."

Mrs. Palmer looked at me and asked, "Yvonne, what do you think about that program?"

I said, "I am sure I could include the music art and PE as part of my day, but Dr. McKnight had told me that I might get too tired, and if I got too tired, I might have to stop going to school. I don't want to stop going to school. Yes, this plan is great! There is nothing I want more than to go to school, play with the kids, and be normal."

The principal looked at my mom and said, "Mrs. Tibbedeaux, what do you think?" Mom replied, "I know how much Yvonne wants to go to school. If it's agreed the one-hour program is a good idea, and all of you are willing to help her, I will do everything I can to make it work. I will walk Yvonne to and from school every day. If after a week Yvonne seems to be strong enough to stay for art or the other electives, I will talk to Mrs. Palmer. If everyone agrees, I will wait and walk her home."

Mrs. Palmer looked at the principal and said, "I think we have a plan." The principal smiled and added, "I think you're right." Then they looked at me and said, "We will see you tomorrow morning."

I looked at Mom. Mom looked at me; we were both crying. I looked at Mrs. Palmer and the principal, and they were crying. Mom thanked Mrs. Palmer and the principal, and I thanked them too. The principal took me by the hand and said she was so pleased I was coming to her school. Mrs. Palmer leaned down and gave me a hug. I loved Mrs. Palmer.

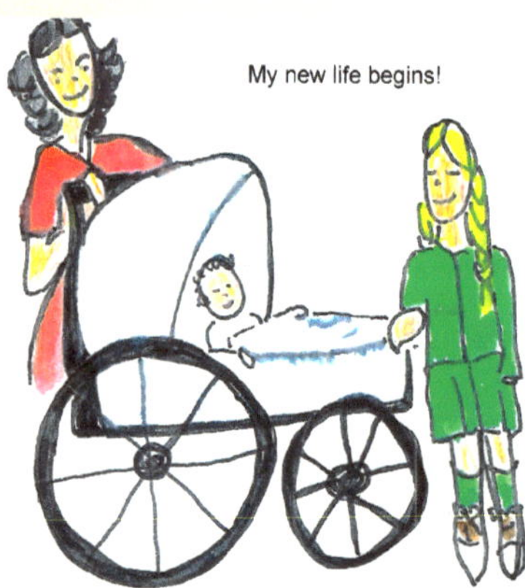

Mom, Donnie, and I walked home from school together. Mom and I talked about how she would walk me to school every day. I wondered if I would need a book bag. What was I going to wear? She had to bring Donnie in the buggy if she was going to walk me to school. Maybe I could walk to school by myself. I had lots of questions, but we were very happy and excited about me going to school.

My new life begins!

Chapter 15

Tyke is ready
for school

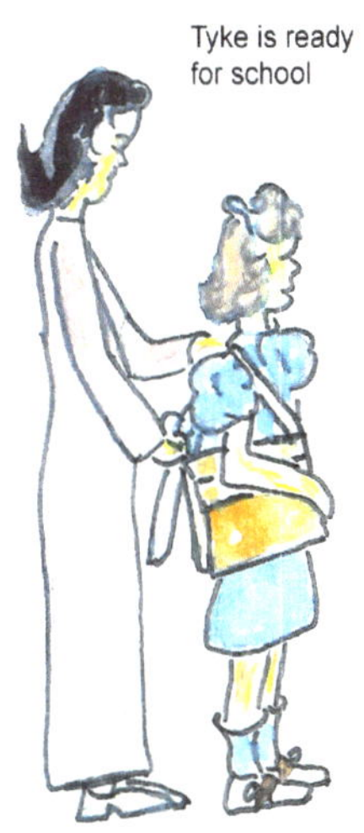

The next morning we got up, Mom and Dad, Donnie, Tyke, and I had breakfast together. Then my sister had to get dressed for school, put her lunch in her lunch pail and her books and papers in her book bag. Mom combed her hair, tied the belt on her dress, and checked to see that she looked just right. Then her girlfriend knocked on our door, and the two girls went off to school. I asked Mom if it was time for me to get dressed for school. She said, "We'll do the dishes, dress the baby, get dressed, then it will be time for us to go." I helped with dishes, made my bed, and got dressed. Mom made me a new dress for the first day of school, and I thought it was pretty. She combed my hair, checked to see if my teeth were brushed and my hand and face were clean. She said, "You look just like a girl on her first day of school. Your dress looks very nice on you." I said, "I love my new dress, Mom. Thanks. Now let's go to school."

I can push Donnie

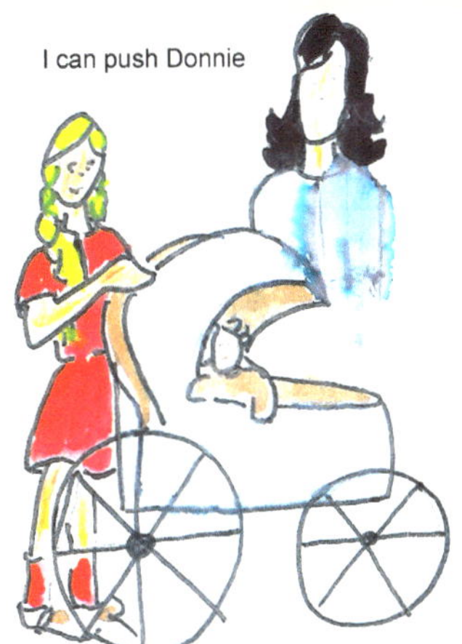

Portola was a small mountain town; most of the streets run up and downhill. The walk to school from our house was not very steep, just a slight incline all the way to the school. I was very excited. I wanted to hurry and get there. I asked Mom if we could push the buggy faster. She said, "We have plenty of time. Your first class doesn't start for fifteen minutes." "But, Mom, we have to go to the principal's office first. Then we have to go find Mrs. Palmer, and she has to take me to the special class. And what if we can't find them, and I'm too late, and I miss my class, I'll have to go home . . ." Mom said, "That isn't going to happen, Yvonne. We have plenty of time. Mrs. Palmer and the principal know we are coming and will be watching for us. You have nothing to worry about."

Going to school that morning was the longest distance I had walked since I had returned home from the hospital. I was beginning to get tired, so I asked Mom if I could push the buggy. She said, "Are you okay? If you're getting tired, we could rest for a minute." I said, "I'm fine. I would just like to rest on the buggy while I'm walking." So Mom let me push the buggy the rest of the way to school.

When we got to the school, there were children all over the playground. I wanted to watch them play. Mom took my hand and led me to the principal's office. The principal and Mrs. Palmer were standing by the door of her office waiting for us.

I am happy
to see you!

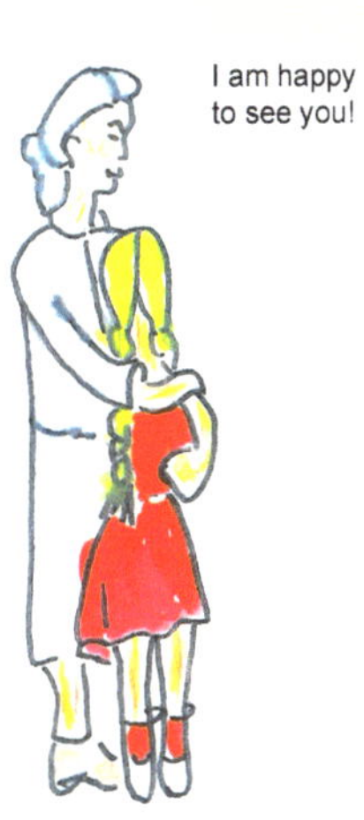

We saw each other at the same time; Mrs. Palmer came toward me with her arms out, and she wrapped them around me in a wonderful welcoming hug. She said she was very happy to see me and that I was right on time. A bell rang, and all the teachers left the hall to get the children from outside. As Mrs. Palmer left, she said she would see me after the special class. The principal said hello to Mom and said Donnie was really cute. Then she looked at me and said, "Are you ready for class?" I answered, "I'm a little scared, but I have waited to be here for a long time, so yes, I'm ready." The principal and I led the way down the hall to the special classroom. Mom and Donnie followed. We waited by the door as the children entered the room. After the children were in the classroom and were sitting down, the principal walked with me over to the teacher's desk and introduced me to the teacher.

Happy to
meet you!

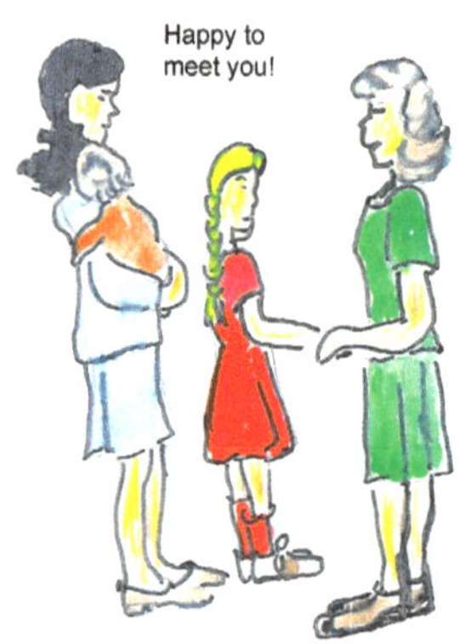

The teacher thanked the principal for bringing me to class and said it was nice to meet me and my mom and baby brother. My mother said she was happy to meet the teacher and see the class. Then she said, "Good-bye. We will meet you at ten thirty in front of the principal's office." I waved good-bye as Mom and Donnie turned and left.

They all looked at me!
A
B

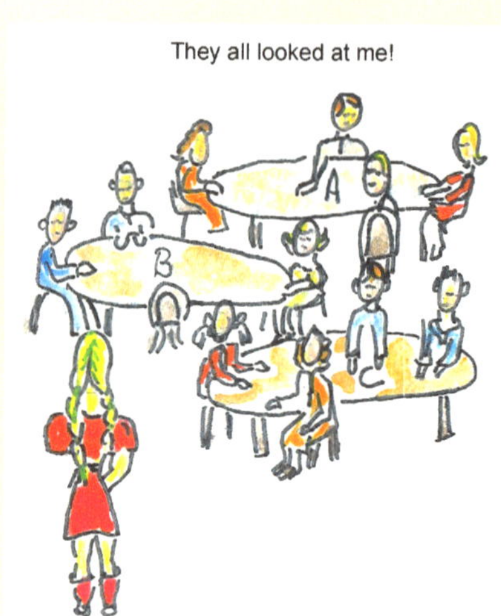

After Mom left, I turned and looked at the class; everybody was looking at me. The teacher said, "I want you to meet Yvonne Tibbedeaux. She is a new student in our class, and she's never been in this school before. I hope that all of you will make her feel welcome."

The teacher asked me to sit at table B. I walked over to a table with *B* written on it and sat in the empty chair. There was a girl and two boys at table B. and they kind of smiled when I sat down. There were four tables in this classroom. It seemed like a very small class to me. There were sixteen children in the class. There were about the same number of boys and girls. The children looked about my size and age.

"Don't cry!"

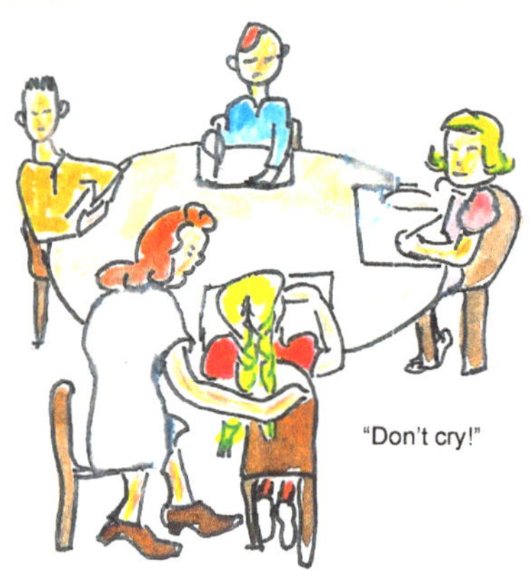

The teacher passed out paper for penmanship practice. There were three lines running across the page to write on; then there was a wide space where you didn't write; then there was another set of three lines to write on. These sets of lines continue down the page. On the first set of lines, we were told to write our first and last names. I wrote *Yvonne.* I didn't know how to write *Tibbedeaux.* I didn't know what to do. All the other kids could write their first and last names. I began to feel sick. I thought I was going to throw up. I put my head on my arm on the table, and I started to cry. The teacher walked over to the table, leaned down, and, in a very soft voice, asked me what was wrong. I told her I didn't know how to write *Tibbedeaux.* She said, "Is that why you're crying?" I nodded my head yes. She said, "Well, of course you can't spell *Tibbedeaux*, I don't think I could spell that name without practice. Today you will begin to learn to spell your very distinctive, beautiful French name, *Tibbedeaux.*" I stopped crying and looked at her; she meant what she said. She wrote my last name on the page next to where I had written *Yvonne. Tibbedeaux* is a very long name. Today I was going to practice so that I could learn how to spell it. I thought she was the best teacher in the world; she understood how some things can be very hard. She had said Tibbedeaux is a beautiful and distinctive name. After penmanship, we had a story. She read a paragraph to the class, and we would read a paragraph quietly to ourselves. Then we would talk to our tablemates about the paragraph we had read. While we were talking to our tablemates about our paragraph, the teacher would come by and talk to us about the words in the paragraph to check if we could pronounce them and if we knew what they meant. We had a word list. A word list was like our own personal dictionary. We wrote the words we needed to know that are new or hard to remember or spell. Then it was time for recess.

Best friends!

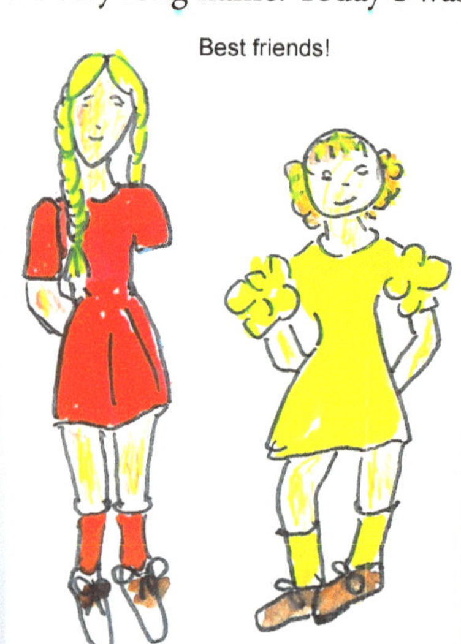

When the teacher dismissed us from class to go to the playground, she asked if the girls at my table would show me around—where to get a drink and where to go to the bathroom. One of the girls at the table said she would like to show me around the school. The girl who said she would help me was Eva Joy. I thought she was the prettiest little girl I had ever seen—she was very small, she had big blue eyes, blonde curly hair, and she liked to smile. When she told me her name was Eva Joy, I thought it was the perfect name for her; she was a joy. She showed me where to get a drink, introduced me to lots of other children, showed me where the bathroom was, and then we played hopscotch. When the bell rang at the end of recess, we went to Mrs. Palmer's class. Eva said, "Mrs. Palmer is the best second grade teacher in the school." Eva and I were both in Mrs. Palmer's class. Then we hugged each other, and she said, "You are my new best friend." I said that she was my best friend too.

Mrs. Palmer took roll call to be sure that all the children were there; she even had my name on the list. Then she said the children going to special class could leave. Eva and I walked to special class together.

The number and the reading classes were located in the same room. The teacher was the same also. Most of the kids were the same, and they sat at the same tables. I was feeling pretty comfortable—I knew the teacher, I had a new friend, I could find my way around the school, and numbers were easy for me. We began the class by counting—first by tens, then five, then two to 100. This was fun. We started at table A then B and C and D. Ten, twenty, thirty . . . then five, ten, fifteen . . . then two, four, six . . . After the oral counting practice, we were asked to write our numbers on the same kind of paper that we'd used to write our name in the earlier class. It was hard work writing all those numbers. I was very tired. I thought I should just put my head down for a minute, and then I'd finish. The next thing I knew, the teacher very quietly told me class was over, and it was time for me to go home. All the other children had gone to recess. She helped me out of the chair, and she took me to the principal's office where my mom and brother were waiting.

Mom looked at me and smiled. "Well, how was your first day at school?" I told her it was great. "I am so tired. Mom, I really worked hard in those classes." The teacher said, "I believe Yvonne had a very good first day. She tried very hard to do everything asked of her. She has a new friend who sits at her table. They played together during recess and learned where the drinking fountain and the bathrooms were located."

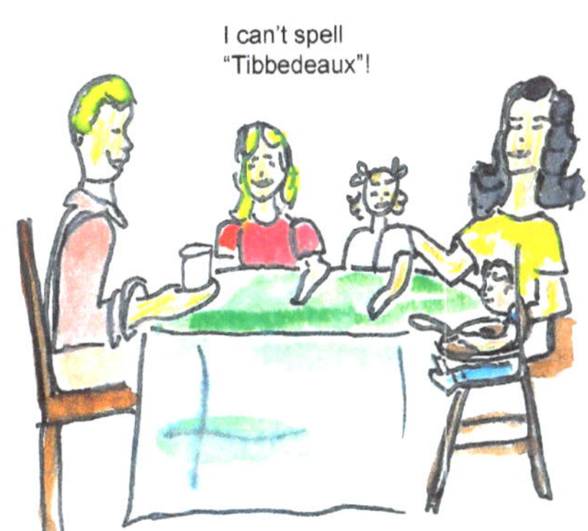

We said good-bye to the teacher and started our walk home. I told Mom it was very important that I learn to write my last name. I told her how bad I felt when everybody could write their last name except me. Mom said she would help me and that I shouldn't feel bad because it's such a long name. Then I told her about Eva Joy and that she said I was her new best friend. She is my best friend also.

By the time we got home, I was so tired I went straight to my bed and lay down. The next thing I knew, Mom was waking me because it was time for dinner. I had slept all afternoon.

At the dinner table that evening, my dad asked me how my first day at school had gone. I told him it was pretty good, but I needed to learn how to spell *Tibbedeaux*. He laughed uproariously; then Mom, Tyke, and I started laughing, and Donnie—who had no idea what we were laughing at—clapped his hands and yelled.

It had been a very good day.

Chapter 16

My first day at school had been a success. I had met my teacher and the principal. I had a girlfriend named Eva. I knew where the classrooms were and how to find my way around the rooms and the school playground.

Waiting for the bell

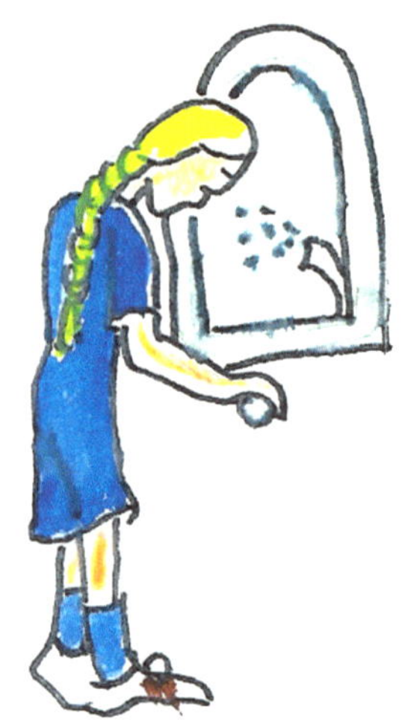

The second day at school, I asked my mom not to walk into the school with me. I didn't need help because I knew where I was going. She gave me a hug, said good-bye, and walked back home with my little brother. As I watched them leave, I felt very free and quite alone. I walked into the school. It was very quiet. Recess had not yet begun, and all the doors to the classrooms were closed. I stood in the hall by myself. I saw the drinking fountain. I decided to get a drink. After I got a drink, I started walking slowly down the hallway. I was waiting for the bell to ring and the doors to open and all the kids to come out of class to go to recess. I walked to the end of the hallway, and then I walked back. The bell still had not rung. I walked down to Mrs. Palmer's classroom and waited. It seemed like I waited a long time, and then finally, the bell rang. Mrs. Palmer was the first one out of the classroom. She held the door open for the children to pass by on their way to the playground. When she saw me, she opened her arms, gave me a hug, and said she was very happy to see me. I felt wonderful! I was so glad I was in school and that Mrs. Palmer was my teacher.

New friends

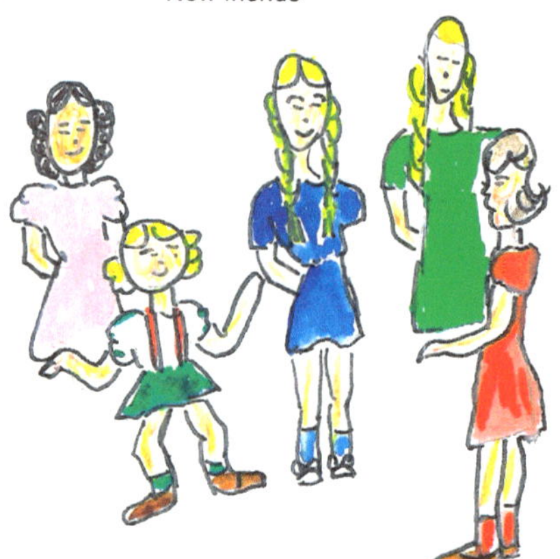

Eva came out of the classroom with some other girls. When she saw me, she said, "I want you to meet my friends." She introduced me to Ann Hecker, Janet Dustan, and Mary Richards. Ann had long blonde braids like mine. I said, "I'm very glad to meet you. My name is Yvonne Tibbedeaux."

Cowgirls

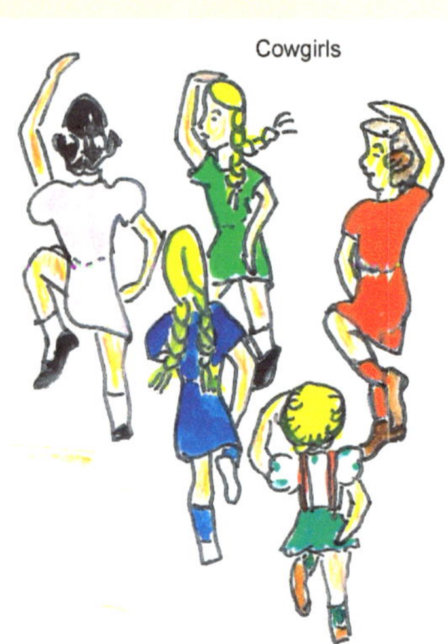

We all walked out to the playground together. Mary said, "Let's play cowgirls." I didn't know how to play cowgirls because I had never played cowgirls before. I decided I would watch and see how they did this because I was sure I could be a cowgirl. As soon as we got to the playground, Mary started trotting and pretended to whip her horse to make it go faster; and Janet, Ann, and Eva did the same thing; and so did I. We raced around the playground as though something was chasing us. Mary was the leader of this cowgirl game. She would tell us we were in terrible danger. We would all scream, run, and hide from the awful danger. It was a wonderful game. We had lots of fun playing cowgirls.

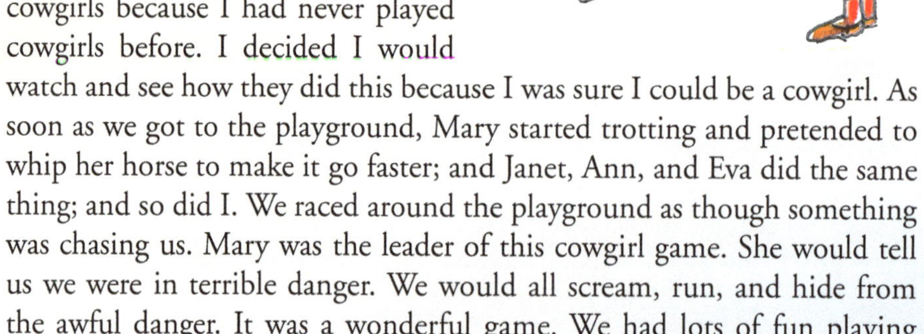

When the bell rang, Janet, Ann, and Mary went to the regular class. Eva and I went to the special reading and language arts class. We said good-bye. We would see each other at the next recess.

We then went to the reading class. The reading teacher said good morning to me, and I told her I was really happy to be back as I took my seat at table B. The teacher asked us to write our first and last name again for penmanship practice. This time, she gave me a paper with my first and last name printed on it. I told her I had practiced writing *Tibbedeaux*, but I still got some of the letters mixed up. I was glad that she gave me a paper with *Tibbedeaux* printed on it. This time, I felt happy and comfortable doing the things she asked me to do. I was doing the same things the other kids were doing. I found out that I could read better than I thought I could. The teacher told me I was doing a very good job. She said my writing was good. I understood about letters and sounds, and I was able to read at a second grade level. She said it was pretty remarkable that I could read second grade level when I had not been in a second grade all year. She made me feel very confident, and that made me feel like an ordinary kid.

My name!

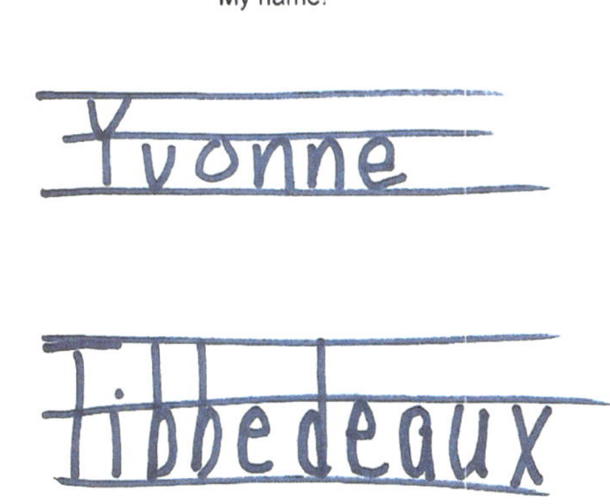

The next recess, Mary, Janet, Ann, Eva, and I played cowgirls again. After recess, we all went back to our regular classes for that period.

After arithmetic class, I said good-bye to Mrs. Palmer and Eva. I went out the front door of the school where my mom and Donnie were waiting. We walked home together, and I told Mom what a great day I had. I had three more new friends who liked to play cowgirl. I told her what a fun game cowgirl is and that Mary had all kinds of good ideas for cowgirls to do. I told her that the teacher said I was doing very well, and I could read at a second grade level. She thought that was good because I had not been in a second grade all year. I asked Mom if I could stay longer tomorrow so I could go to art or music or PE class. She said she would think about it, and she would talk to the principal tomorrow.

When I got home, I was very tired and very happy. Mom and Donnie and I had lunch, and I lay down and went to asleep. When I woke, Tyke was home from school, my dad was home from work, and dinner was on the table. We all talked about our day at dinner. My sister was having a good time at school. She had lots of friends, and she was a good student. I told Daddy and my sister all the fun things I had done at school, and I hoped I would be able to stay for the art and PE classes. Mom said she would talk to the principal and Mrs. Palmer tomorrow, but I probably wouldn't stay tomorrow because I still needed to rest at the end of that hour. She said, "Today is Tuesday, and you are less tired today than you were yesterday. Maybe you can stay on Friday of this week." I was disappointed, but I didn't argue because I knew Mom was right. I'd been pretty tired at the end of the hour of classes today.

Wednesday morning, Mom, Donnie and I walked to school. We went to the principal's office. It was agreed that I would stay for PE on Friday after my arithmetic class. I would come home from school one-half hour later on Friday.

Each day I became more confident and comfortable I felt more healed than I had for a long time. I was a normal kid. I was going to school. I had friends and I had teachers that I loved. Now I was going to be able to play games at school during PE. I couldn't wait for Friday.

Friday morning finally came. We walked to school as usual. I said good-bye to Mom and Donnie at the door. I went to Mrs. Palmer's class to meet Eva, and we went to recess and then to reading class. After reading class, we had another recess; we played with all our girlfriends. After recess, we went to arithmetic class, and after that class, we went to another recess and then to PE.

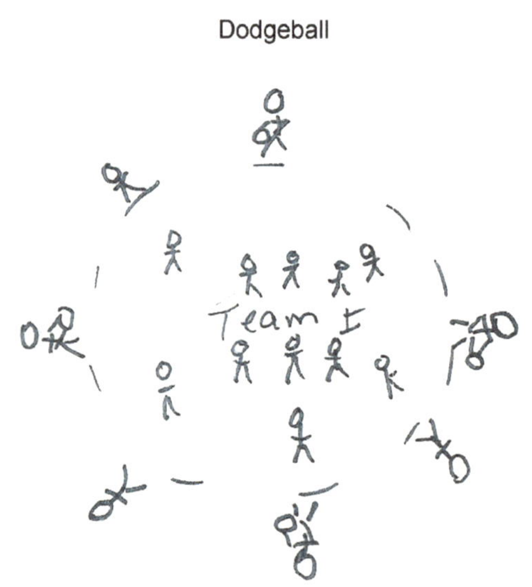

We all got together on the playground with a PE teacher. "Today we are going to play dodgeball. The way we play dodgeball is to have two teams, and the teams are chosen by making a big circle and then counting one then two all around the circle." The ones stepped into the circle. That was one team. The two stepped back five paces. That was the other team. The outside circle had to throw the ball at the team inside of the circle. The object of the game was for the outside circle people to hit the inside circle people with the ball. When all the inside circle people were hit, and out of the game, the outside circle people had to go inside the circle. The game then started all over. The rules were that the ball was never to be thrown higher than the knee, and the ball should not be thrown hard. A fast rolling ball was the proper throw. I was on team one, so I had to step into the circle. The balls were going to be thrown at me and my team. My job was to try to avoid the ball so I wouldn't get hit by the ball and have to leave the game.

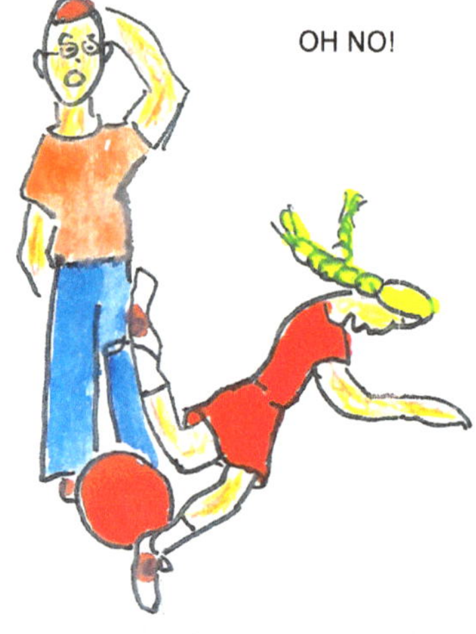

The kids on team two threw the ball. On the first throw, four kids in the circle were hit by the ball. They had to leave the center of the circle. They were out of the game. The ball missed me. I was still in the game. Several more throws were made, and more kids were out of the game. I was still in the game. No one had hit me yet. One of the boys from team two threw the ball very hard right at me and knocked me down. Everybody gasped. I had fallen hard. The boy who threw the ball that knocked me down came to me and said he was very sorry. He said he didn't mean to knock me down. I said, "That's okay. I'm fine." I got up from the ground. I had scraped my knee and my arm and both were bleeding. The PE teacher told the boy, who threw the ball that hit me, to take me to the nurse's office. Douglas Joy was the boy who knocked me down. He was Eva's cousin. He felt bad about hurting me. I told him it didn't hurt that bad. He said he was still sorry. He walked into the nurse's office where she cleaned the scratches and put Band-Aids on my wounds. By the time we got back to the playground, team two was in the circle, and team one was throwing the ball. Douglas got in the circle, and I got to throw the ball. I liked being in PE class, and I liked getting to meet Douglas Joy.

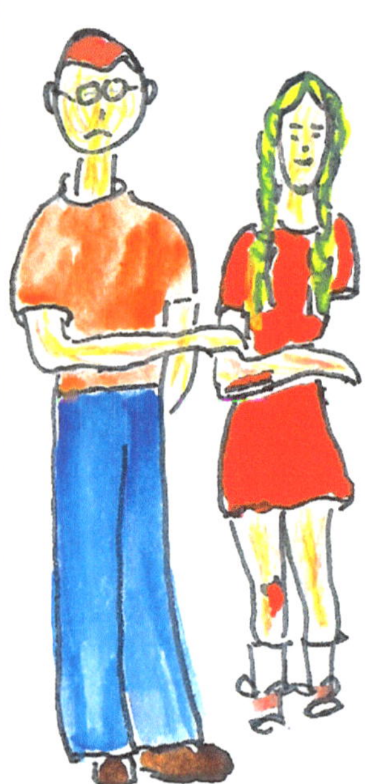

After PE, most of the kids went to lunch. I met Mom and Donnie at the front door of the school. Mom saw my Band-Aids and wanted to know what happened to me. I told her that we played dodgeball during PE, and Douglas threw the ball too hard, hit me, and I fell down. The teacher told Douglas to take me to the nurse's office where the nurse washed my arm and knee and put on the Band-Aids. Mom said that dodgeball is kind of a rough game. She asked if I was mad at Douglas for knocking me down. I said, "I think he is a really nice boy, and he didn't mean to hurt me." I was not mad at him.

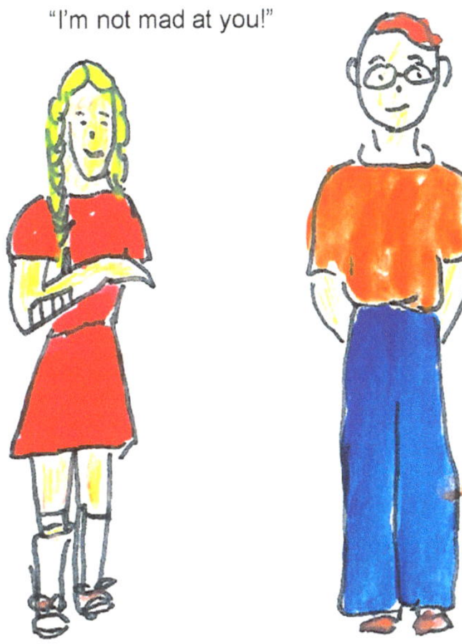

The first week of school was over. It had been a very successful return to school for me. Mom had met with the principal and Mrs. Palmer when I was in PE class. It was decided that I could go to music, art, story time, and PE after arithmetic class. It would lengthen my day by one-half hour. One-half hour is not a lot of time, but it was proof that I was getting better, and I could manage just fine in school.

I am back in the game!

Chapter 17

Being back in school even for an hour and a half a day was very successful in making me feel like a regular kid doing regular things at school. The routine of walking to school with my mother and little brother, seeing my friends at recess and playing games with them, going to special reading class and special arithmetic class, and the activity classes of art, music, story, or PE was exactly the therapy I needed. I was feeling good and ready for the next step.

My one-and-one-half hour school schedule continued for a week. At the end of the week, my mother and I met with the principal and Mrs. Palmer. This time, we asked if I could come to school in the morning at the beginning of the school day and stay through lunch. This would increase my day by one hour. The best part about this, for me, was that I would be able to walk to school with my sister and other children instead of having my mother take me. Having lunch with the other students would be a special treat for me and would provide more time for socializing with my friends. Mrs. Palmer supported the idea. She said she would enjoy having me in her class at the beginning of the day. She also said one other benefit to this schedule was that if I was tired at lunchtime, I could leave early and have lunch at home. The principal wanted to know who would walk me home. My mother said she thought I could walk home by myself. There was some discussion between the adults about whether or not I could walk home alone especially if I was tired. I said I didn't think I would be too tired to walk home by myself. The principal said she really did not like children walking home alone without specific times for their leaving school and arriving at home. My mother said that she and my brother could come at lunchtime and wait for me. The principal said she had no objections to me staying if my mom was willing to meet me at school.

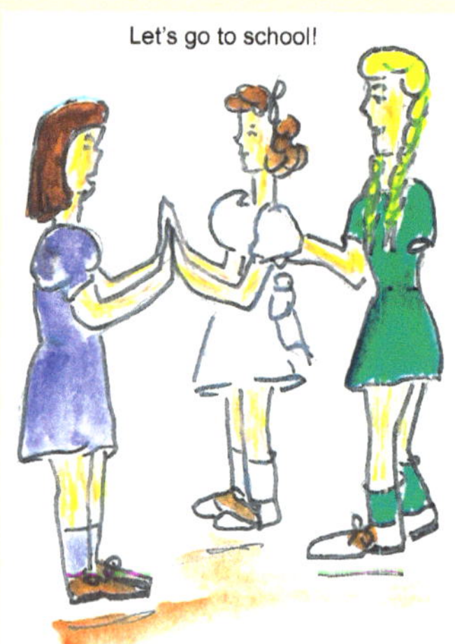

Starting the third week, I would be able to come to school when school started in the morning and stay until after lunch. I really wanted to walk home by myself, but I was not going to complain about this compromise. On our way home from school that morning, I told my mother she was the best friend any kid could have. I also told her that I knew it was a lot of work for her and Donnie to come and meet me at school every day. She told me that the exercise was good for her, and Donnie loved to go for walks. She was the greatest mom in the world, and my heart ached with all the love I felt for her that day.

Walking to school in the morning with other kids was a great way to start my day. There were kids walking to school from kindergarten all the way to sixth grade. The boys ran around, punching each other and teasing the girls. The girls giggled and pretended they hated the boys. My sister introduced me to all her friends, and we talked and laughed about all the things little girls talk and laugh about.

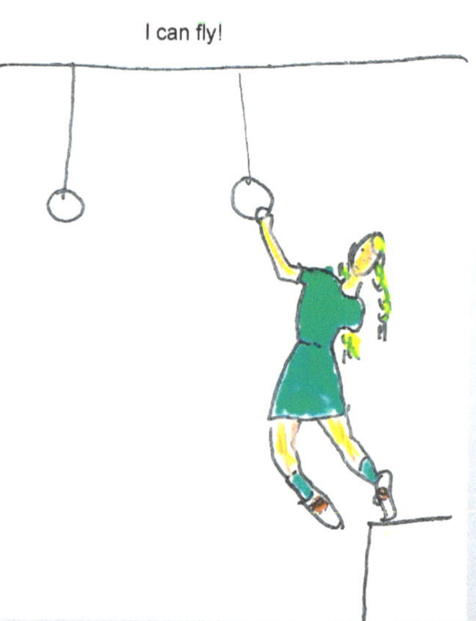

When we got to school, we went straight to the playground. We put our lunch pails, books, and sweaters in a pile near the classroom door. I always liked to play on the rings, the monkey bars, and climbing bar. I liked to hang on the ring, step up on the platform, push off, and go as far as I could in the air. One day, I lost my grip on the ring and

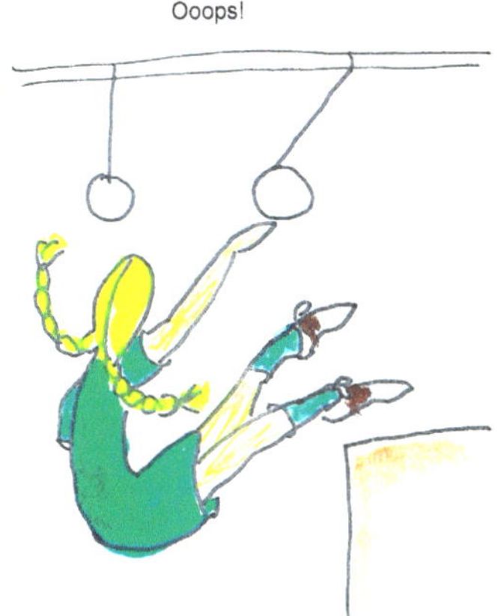

fell. I didn't get hurt. I got right back up and grabbed the ring and prepared to push off again. Just before I pushed off, the yard teacher came over and told me I couldn't play on the rings. I asked her why. She said it was too dangerous for me. I said all the other kids play on the rings. She said yes, but they had two arms and I didn't. I said it didn't take two arms to swing on the ring. I could do it with one. She told me I was a very rude child, and she was taking me to the principal's office. I was furious. When we got to the principal's office, the teacher said that I had been rude and disrespectful to her. The principal looked at her and at me and said, "What did you do, Yvonne?" I told her that the teacher told me that I couldn't play on the rings because I only had one arm. I told the principal that I tried to explain to the teacher that I could play on the rings with one arm because it didn't take two arms to play on the rings. The teacher told me I was being rude, and she was going to bring me to you. That's what happened.

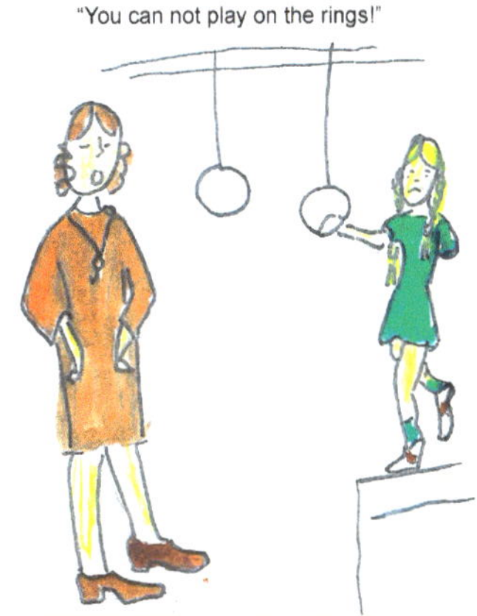

The principal said to the teacher that she didn't understand. The teacher said, "Yvonne forgot to mention that she had just fallen off the ring. The rings are high and obviously too dangerous for this child to be on them." The principal asked the teacher what I had done to her that was rude. The teacher felt that I had been rude when I said that I could play on the rings with one arm. I said that because I'd been playing on the rings for several days, and I hadn't fallen before, and I wasn't hurt. I was just trying to explain to her that it could be done with one arm.

The principal told me to stay off the rings until she could investigate to find out if the rings were a danger or were a proper apparatus for me to play on. I was shocked. I didn't think I had done anything wrong. I thought the yard teacher had been rude to me. "How dare she tell me that I can't play on things because I have one arm." This was not fair. She didn't know anything about having one arm, or what I could or couldn't do, or why I should or shouldn't do it. I thought she was unkind, rude, but most of all, she was ignorant. I didn't say any of these things, but I was so angry I cried. I didn't want that yard teacher to see me cry. I turned around so she couldn't see me and started to walk out of the principal's office. The principal said, "Yvonne, I need to talk to you. Please wait a minute." I stopped by the door. After the yard teacher left the office, I turned around. I was still crying. I didn't want the principal to see me cry. So I looked at the floor. She asked me to please sit down. She sat down next to me. She said she was sorry that my feelings were hurt. She said, "I need you to understand that everyone at the school is concerned about you and wants you to do well." She explained, "It's impossible for us to have any idea of how hard it must be for a little girl, eight years old, to deal with all the problems that you have had to deal with. You are so brave. You lost your arm. You nearly lost your life because of gas gangrene, a deadly infection. You were a trial case for a new and unproved drug.

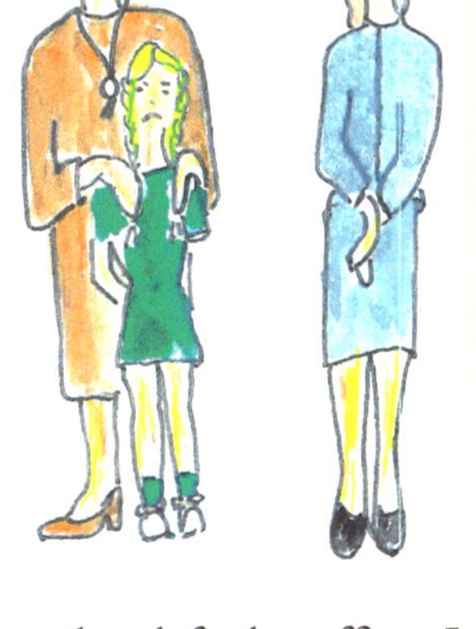

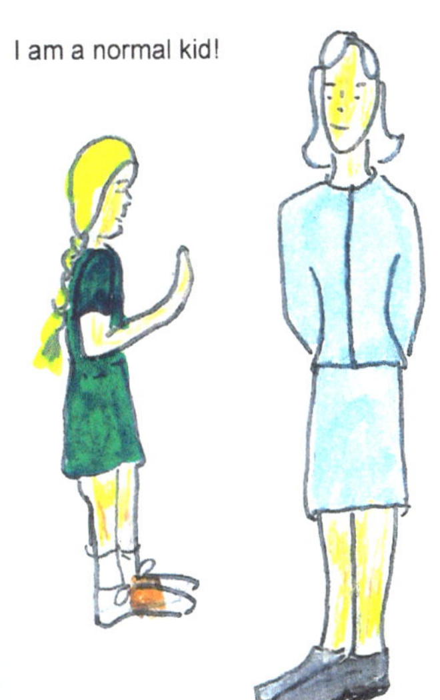

You became addicted to morphine, the drug that was used to keep the pain under control. You lost more than half of your body weight. You were so weak that you could not walk. You wore big bulky bandages for months because the wound caused by the amputation and residual infection would not heal. You had to go and stay alone hundreds of miles away from home, to a hospital in San Francisco, for surgery so that your arm would heal and you could stop wearing bandages. You have triumphed over impossible odds, and in less than a month after your last surgery, you started coming to school. You were so weak and so unwell it took all the strength you had to stay at school for one-half hour. Every week you pushed to work harder and stay longer. You have been in school less than a month, and you are attending half a day. You have asked for no special privileges. You have asked for no special help. You are doing and have done everything your teachers have asked you to do. You have friends. You have had a few scrapes, and now a fall from the rings. At no time did you ever complain about being tired or sick. All you have ever asked from us is to treat you like a normal kid. The truth is you are so far from normal that we tend to want to help and protect you. I'm beginning to understand that for you, the best help we can offer is to let you figure it out, whatever the problem."

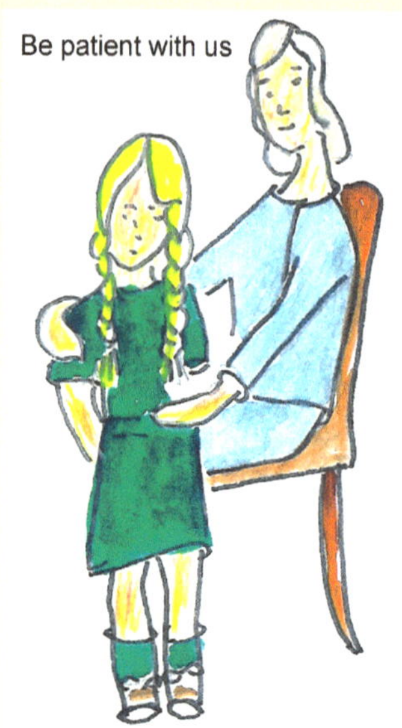

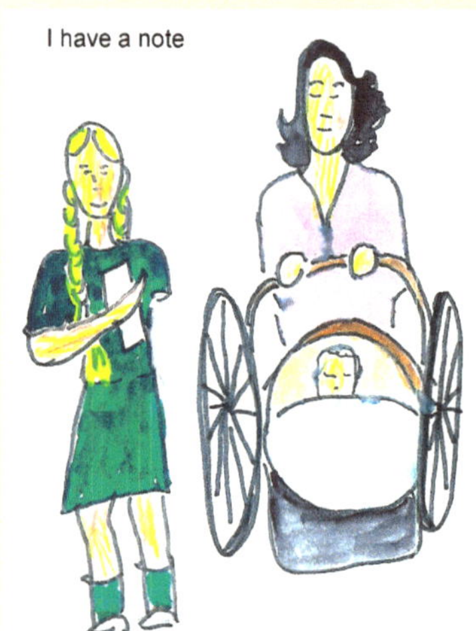

Then she said, "I know you're very angry with the yard teacher. She should not have said that you cannot play on the rings because you have one arm. What she should have said, and what I think she meant, is that she thought they weren't safe because you can easily slip off the rings and get hurt. When you came in this morning to my office, I said that I would investigate to see if the rings are safe for you to play on. That is what I intend to do. Whatever my decision, it will be made in your best interest, in so far as I understand the situation. I hope that you will be patient with us. We don't want you to get hurt. We want you to be able to do anything you can safely do. I will send a letter home with you to give to your mother." Then she said to me, "Do you think you can forgive the yard duty teacher?" I said, "I can forgive her for telling me not to play on the rings. But it will be very hard for me to forgive her for saying it is because I have one arm that I cannot play on the rings." Then to the principal I said, "All I want to be is a normal kid who can do normal things where ever I am."

Fairness is not a right.

Chapter 18

Let's go see Dr. McKnight.

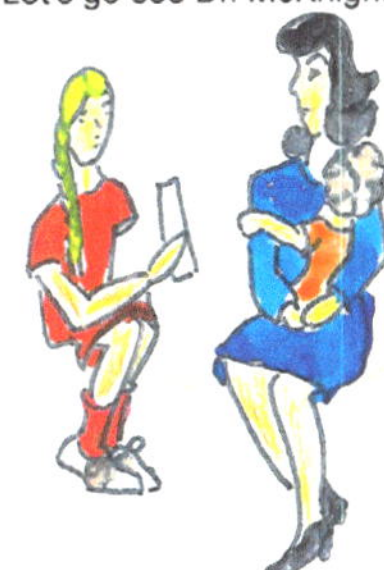

When I left the principal's office, my mother was waiting for me in front of the school. I was still crying and very angry. She asked me why I was crying. I handed her the letter. Mom sat down on a bench by the front of the school and read the letter. Then she looked at me and said, "We need to talk to Dr. McKnight." I asked her what the letter said, and she told me, "The principal needed some guidelines about what is safe for you to play on at school. She also said that you would not be allowed to play on any structure until we had set the rules."

I thought I was doing great!

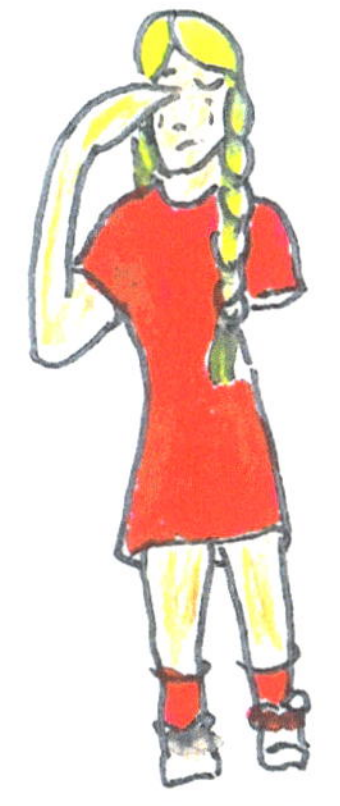

I started crying again because I was so angry and so disappointed and hurt. I thought things had been going very well in school. I didn't know that the teachers were all worried about me and afraid I would get hurt if I acted like normal kids and played on the school playground equipment. I thought I was a normal kid, and now I wasn't sure.

Mom said, "Let's walk to Dr. McKnight's office right now and ask him what he thinks our guidelines should be. We need to talk about how you should be treated." Should there be a special set of rules for a handicapped child? I told Mom I thought that it would be a good idea to help the teachers understand that I was a normal kid. My mother, my brother, and I walked to Dr. McKnight's office.

"You are a normal kid
with a handicap"

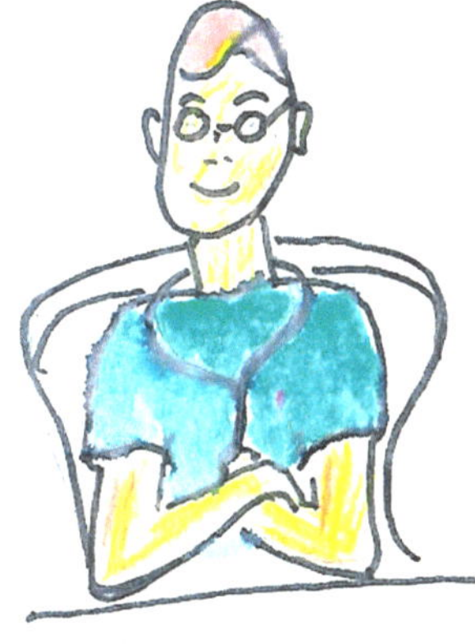

When Dr. McKnight saw us at his office, he smiled and said how happy he was to see us. Then he looked at me closely and said, "What's the matter? Have you been crying?"

Mom told Dr. McKnight that I had a bad day at school and that if he had time, we would like to talk to him about the problem. He told us he always had time to talk with us to try to solve problems. He invited us into his private office where we sat down around a table so we could talk. Mom handed Dr. McKnight the letter from the principal. He read the letter, put it down on the table, and looked right at me. He told me that I could play on any apparatus at school or any place else that I felt comfortable and able to manage. He said the risk of getting hurt was the same for me as it was for any other child. Every child who played on an apparatus could get hurt. "Your arm is healed, Yvonne. You are always going to have one arm, and you have to figure out what you can do. If you fall and you're not hurt, get up and go play. If you have a scratch, get a Band-Aid. If you break something, come and see me, and I'll fix it. I would give this advice to any child going to school, to a park, a swimming pool, hiking up a hill, walking on logs, or just running and playing. You are a normal child with a handicap. There is no reason why you shouldn't be able to do whatever you think is safe for you. You are a child, however, and you need to follow the rules and guidelines set by the school."

Mom asked the doctor if he'd noticed the last sentence in the letter. He said, "You mean where it says that you need to write a letter, taking full responsibility for your daughter's actions at school and on the playground?" Mom said yes and asked him what would happen if Yvonne got hurt at school. "What does it mean that the parents are held responsible for what happens to their child?" The doctor said, "The parent is always responsible for their child's behavior. The school wants you to take responsibility in a written form, simply means that you cannot sue them if Yvonne gets hurt on any apparatus in good repair at school."

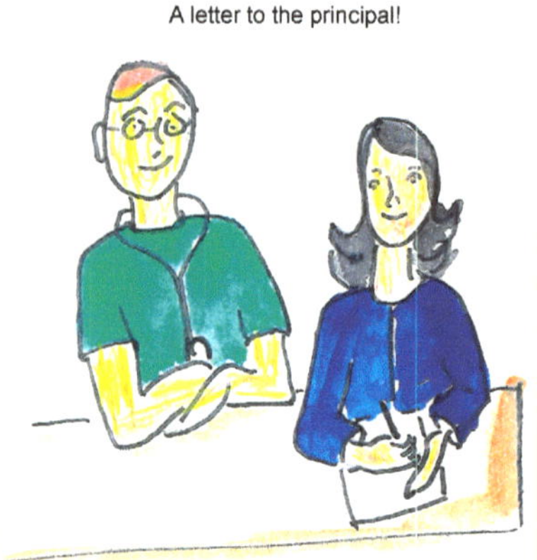
A letter to the principal!

While Donnie and I sat and waited, Dr. McKnight and Mom wrote a letter to the principal:

Yvonne's father and I are very appreciative of the effort and time that you and your staff have given to Yvonne in order for her to enter school on a very special schedule due to her health concerns. There is no question that you and the teachers are helping Yvonne in so many ways to gain self-confidence in her ability to read and write, to do arithmetic and numbers, to meet and play with children. You willingly altered your schedule to meet her needs. As she gets healthier, she can stay longer and do more. Your concern for Yvonne's safety at school is most appropriate. As Yvonne's parents, we are also concerned about her well-being. After reading the letter you sent home with Yvonne, her father and I had a conversation with Dr. McKnight, who is convinced that there is no reason why Yvonne cannot do anything at school she feels comfortable doing within the rules. The doctor assures us that she is healed and in no more danger than any other child at school. Yvonne is a perfectly normal child with a handicap. Working with a handicapped child is new for all of us. Our experience has been that Yvonne tends to push herself. She is impatient to do all the things she hasn't been able to do because of illness. We believe that your concerns are honest, helpful, and appropriate. We also believe that Yvonne is going to need every bit of the courage and determination she can muster to deal with her handicap.

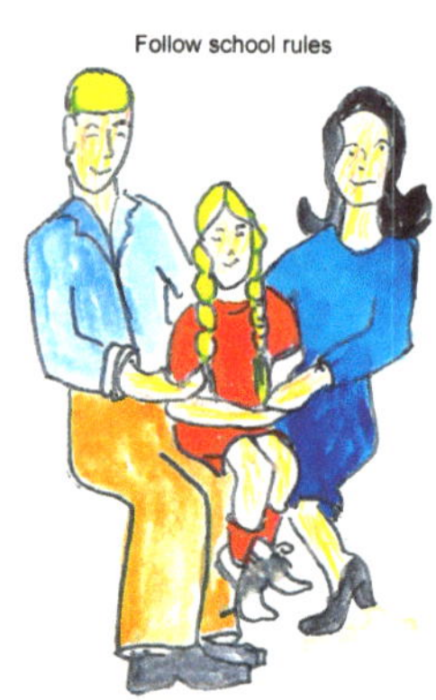
Follow school rules

That evening, after Daddy got home, he and Mom talked for a long time about the letter. My dad thought it was a good letter, and he and Mom finished the letter by saying that they would meet with the principal and any teachers who wanted to talk about how to keep me safe and still encourage me to try to do things that were hard to watch a one-armed child do. They did not want special rules for me. They expected me to follow the rules of the school. They felt that there was no need for special one-armed child rules. They said they would take full responsibility for normal playing at school, including the use of school playground apparatus. My parents both signed the letter.

The next day, when my mother came to meet me at school, she went to talk to the principal. She gave her the letter. They made an appointment for my father and mother to meet with the staff involved with my activities at school. The day and time for the meeting was arranged. And a few days later, they met. I was not invited to go to the meeting.

After the meeting, Mom and Dad told me that I was very lucky to be going to school where the teachers and the principal and all the people who worked with me were trying so hard to help me. They told me it was my responsibility to follow the rules of school. If I felt that something wasn't fair, I was to tell them about it. I was not to argue with the teacher about anything. I told them that I thought they were great for talking to the teachers and that there would be no one-armed child rules on the playground.

Fairness was worth fighting for!

Chapter 19

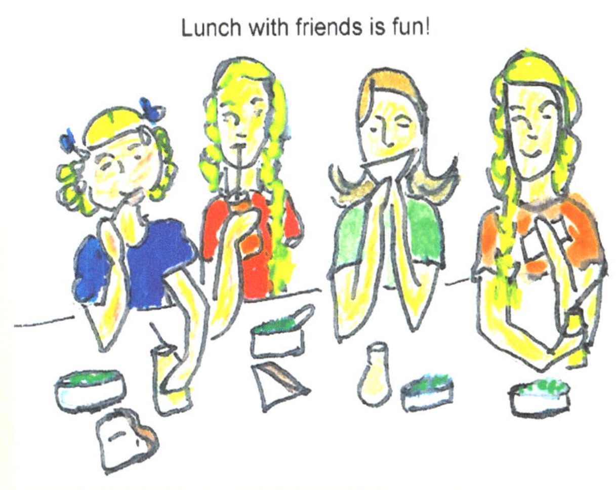
Lunch with friends is fun!

The day after my parents' meeting with the school staff, I went back to school to my special schedule and played on the playground apparatus, including the rings. I also played cowgirls with my friends and ate lunch at school and walked home with Mom and Donnie. I was a normal kid doing normal things.

The following week, beginning on Monday, I went to school at the beginning of the day. I had lunch with my class in the cafeteria. I went to afternoon classes and walked home with all the other kids at the end of the day. It was the first time in two years that I spent all day at school. I felt a little tired but wonderful.

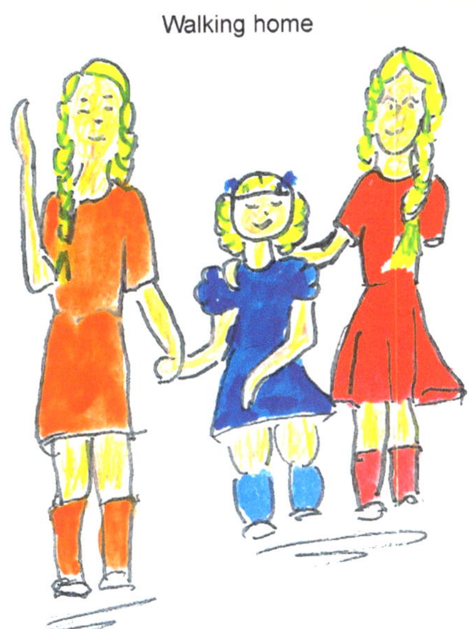
Walking home

The children going to school in Portola in 1944 brought their lunch (usually a sandwich) to eat at school. Milk and a hot dish, usually vegetable soup, or just plain cooked vegetables was provided by the school as part of the children's lunch. The children were expected to drink the milk and eat the vegetables provided by the school. Some teachers were very strict about this and insisted that every child in their class eat everything provided.

I was very pleased and happy to be able to go to school all day. I liked Mrs. Palmer and the special reading and math teacher.

The teacher that walked our class to lunch was also the teacher that took me to the principal's office when I fell off the rings. For some reason, she didn't like me. I tried very hard to be polite to her and do everything she asked me to do because I didn't want any more problems at school. She would single me out each day to walk next to her as we walked to the cafeteria. You may think she did that because she liked me, but that's not why she did it. She walked next to me to be sure I didn't make a mistake.

About a week into this new program, I came to school, and I didn't feel very well. I told Mrs. Palmer that I felt sick. She thought maybe if I ate my lunch, I would feel better. I told her I would try. When Mrs. Palmer met with the lunch teacher, she mentioned to her that I had said I felt unwell and might not be able to eat lunch. The lunch teacher directed me to walk next to her, which I did. I told her I didn't feel good. As we walked down the hall, I could smell creamed peas, and then I really felt terrible. I told her that I thought I was going to be sick. The creamed peas' smell made me nauseous. The lunch teacher said, "You will eat lunch, and you will eat cream peas." I wanted to tell her that I didn't think I should because I really felt sick. I didn't want to get in trouble, so I didn't say any more. I was afraid she would take me to the principal again if I told her that I couldn't eat the peas.

When we got into the cafeteria, the lunch teacher told all the children where to sit. She told me to sit next to her. I was feeling really sick. I thought I was going to throw up. I sat back in my chair and tried

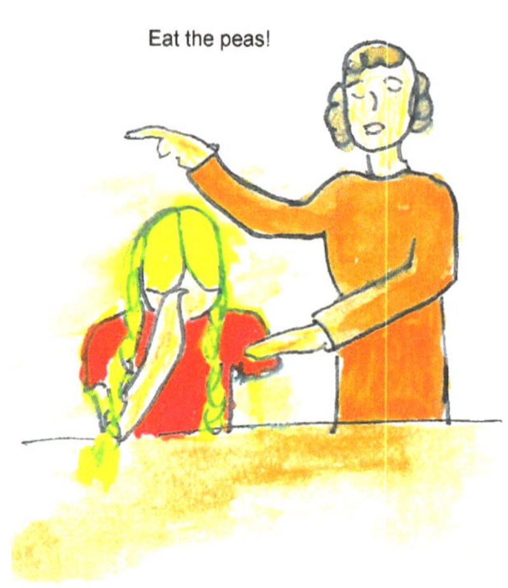

to put my head down in my lap. The lunch teacher directed me to sit up and eat the creamed peas first. I put a spoonful in my mouth, and I started to gag. The teacher became enraged, and she yelled at me to stop that and eat the peas. I tried to take another bite, and I threw up all over her, the table, myself, and another child. She jumped up from the table and screamed at me. I got out of my chair and ran out of the cafeteria as fast as I could. I ran outside. I threw up about four more times on the way to the wall. There was a low wall encircling the school. I climbed over the wall, threw up several more times, and lay down on the ground. My head ached, and my stomach hurt. I felt hot and sweaty, and I was shivering. I heard the lunch teacher calling me, but I didn't want her to know where I was. I didn't say a word. I just lay on the ground by the wall with my eyes closed.

The school in Portola was in the middle of a neighborhood. There were houses all around the school. It never occurred to me that while I was lying on the ground with my eyes closed—and feeling very sick—some of the school's neighboring homeowners were watching me. I was too sick to care. The only thing I wanted was to be left alone. I was so sick, and I didn't want her to find me.

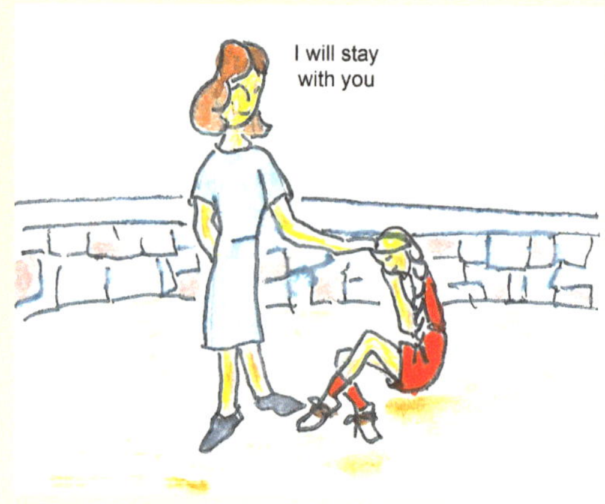

A lady across the street from where I was lying down saw me and came over to see if she could help. In the meantime, another person who was home and saw me lying on the ground called the school and told the principal there was a sick child throwing up by the wall in front of school grounds. I told the lady who came over to help me that I was too sick to get up or move. She said she would stay with me until someone came to help. About this time, the lunch teacher saw the lady sitting by the wall, and she walked over to ask why she was there, and then she saw me lying on the ground. The principal also came over by the wall to see which child was lying on the ground sick.

The lunch teacher came over the wall and said, "What in the world are you doing here?" I told her I was sick and to please leave me alone. She told me I had to get up from the ground because it was cold and wet. I told her I was afraid I'd get sick again if I moved too much. She said she would help me get up and walk me back to the school office. I started to cry. I did not want to go to the principal's office and be in trouble again. It wasn't my fault. I was sick. By this time, the principal had joined the little group by the wall. She asked me why I was crying. I told her that I was very embarrassed because I got sick in the cafeteria, and I threw up all over everybody. I told her I really felt very sick, and I just wanted to go home.

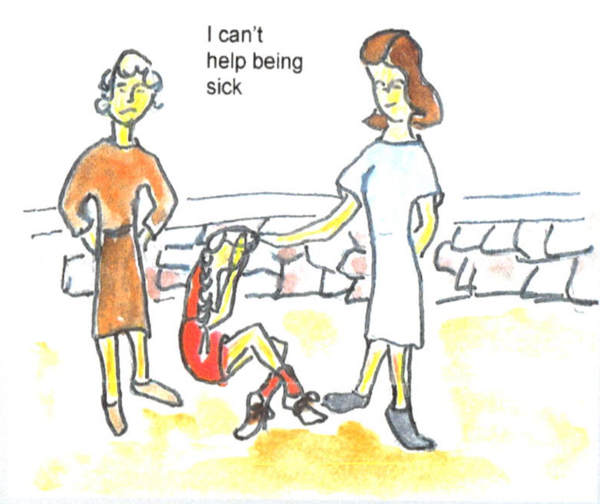

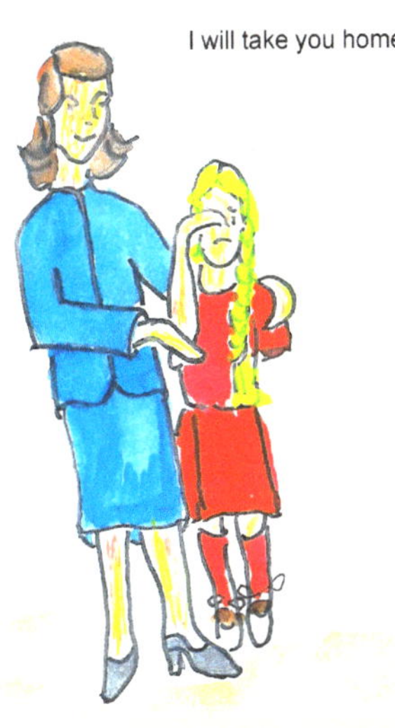

The principal asked the lunch teacher why she made me stay in the cafeteria when I was obviously sick. She said she didn't know I was sick. She thought I was just trying to get out of eating the creamed peas, which were an important part of the lunch.

The principal gently lifted me up from the ground, put her arm around me, and said, "Please don't cry, Yvonne. I can see that you are sick. I'll take you home."

There is still a lot of work to do!

Chapter 20

After the principal took me home from school, she and Mom had a long talk about how things were going for me at school. The principal felt that I had made remarkable progress. She was concerned that I was pushing myself too hard and was perhaps trying too hard to please everyone at school in order to be accepted as a normal child. My mother agreed and thought I was overstressed and tired. She thought that might have been the reason I got sick at school. Mom told the principal that she would keep me home for a day or two until I was feeling better.

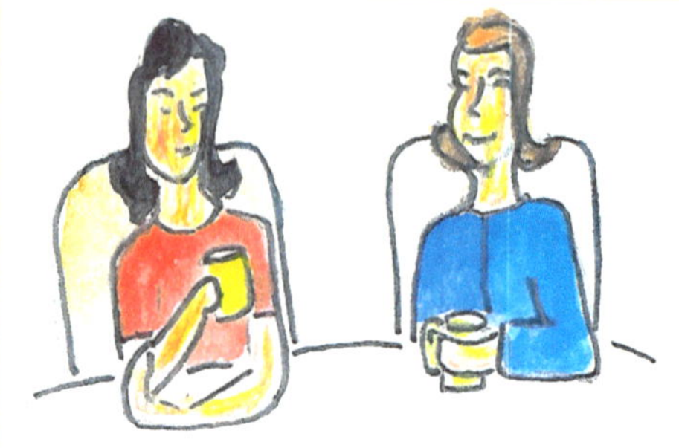

Yvonne is trying too hard

By the time Mom and the principal had finished their conference, I was sound asleep. Later that afternoon, she told me she thought I needed to stay home from school for a few days until I was feeling better. I told her that I was feeling fine now. I was sure I would be ready for school tomorrow morning. She said, "We will see how you are feeling in the morning."

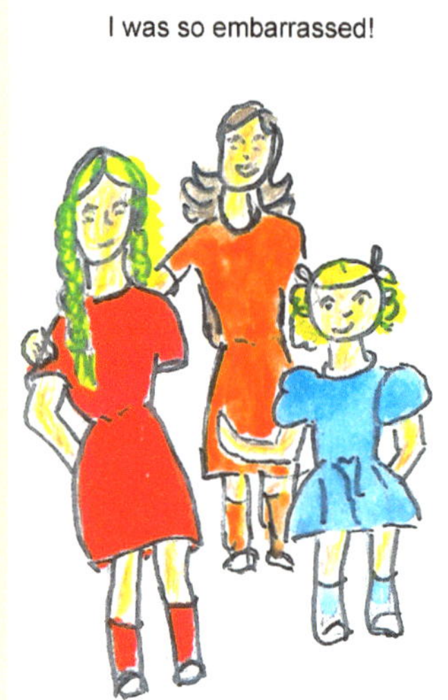

I was so embarrassed!

That evening, I didn't feel well enough to eat dinner. My stomach still felt funny. The next day, I did stay home from school and slept most of the day. By the following day, I felt better and went to school.

I was dreading seeing the teachers and the kids when I got back to school because I really was embarrassed about getting sick in the cafeteria. But all my friends were happy to see me, and nobody said anything about me being sick in the cafeteria.

I had been in school now for almost two months. My school day had changed from one hour a day to a full primary school day. I had made friends. My schoolwork was average. The whole school was aware that I was a perfectly normal kid with a handicap. I was happier, healthier, and more self-confident than any of us had expected.

May was the last month of school, and a special program was going to be presented for the parents. It was a Mother's Day program presented by all the classes in the school. I don't remember what the upper classes did for the program. I was in second grade, and Tyke was in first grade. Both classes were going to sing lullabies with an international theme. The lullabies were going to be sung by all of the children in the two classes. Four girls in the second grade class were selected to act as mothers rocking their babies while the lullabies, representing each country, were being sung. Mrs. Palmer asked if there was anyone in our class who is French. I raised my hand and said I was French. Mrs. Palmer asked if I could dress up like a French mother and bring my baby doll wrapped in a blanket to rock in a rocking chair while the chorus sang a French lullaby. I said I would love to do that. So I became the French mother in our school program. Three other girls were chosen to represent other countries as mothers for the Mother's Day program.

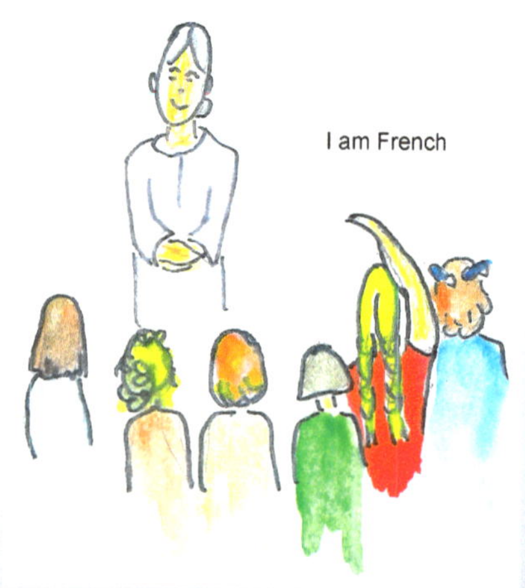

I am French

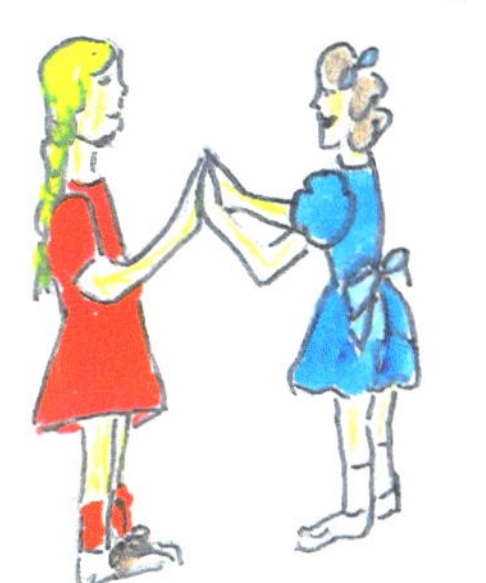

That day, as we walked home from school, we were so excited because we were in the program. Tyke said that I was the star of the program. But really the stars of the program were the singers because they made the music for the show. The girls who played the mothers were just a backdrop for the music, but I was excited about dressing up like a French mother and rocking my doll in front of everybody.

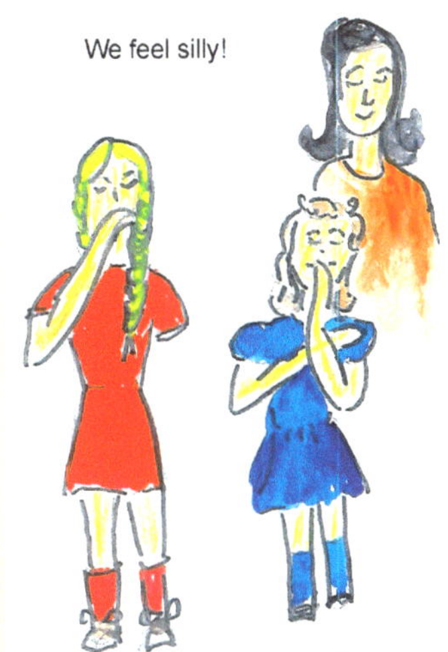

When we got home that day, my sister and I came running into the house to tell Mom that she had to make me a French mother's costume. And I would need one of Donnie's baby blankets to wrap up my doll. Tyke was in first grade. First and second grades were the singers. The singers needed to dress up in their nicest clothes. Because Tyke was small and had a very good voice, she got to stand in the front row of all the singers. We were both very excited and silly about being in the program.

We told Mom we were in the program. Tyke was a singer in the front row and needed to wear a pretty dress, and I was the French mother, and I needed a French mother's dress and a baby wrapped in a blanket. Mom wanted to know what a French mother wore. I looked at Tyke; she looked at me. We started to giggle and then laughed until tears ran down our cheeks. Mom asked, "What is so funny?" It took a minute for us to be able to respond. Then we told her we had no idea. All three of us started laughing about being so excited about something we had no idea about.

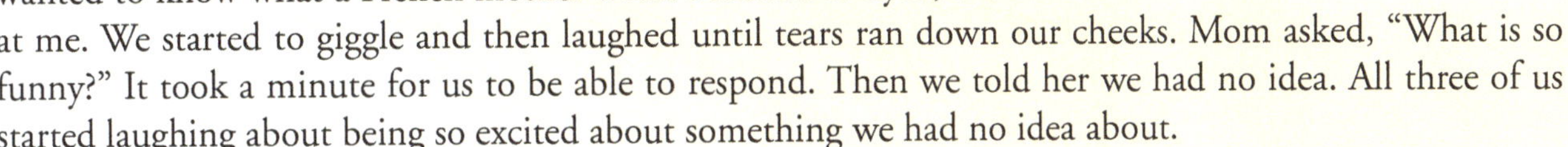

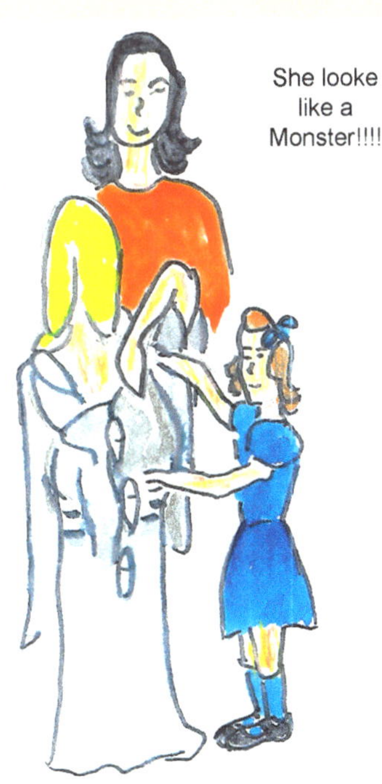

Luckily, Mom knew just what a French mother would wear. She went to her closet and found an old black dress she was planning to give away. She helped me try it on. The dress was way too long so she got an old belt, tied it around my waist, and we pulled the top up until we could see my feet. Now the dress was short enough but was much too big around. She told us not to worry, and she pinned the back with some of Donnie's diaper pins. Tyke looked at me. I looked at her. We started to shake our heads; then we grinned and started to giggle and laugh. Mom wanted to know what was so funny. Tyke said, "Yvonne looks like a Halloween monster all pinned together." We all started laughing.

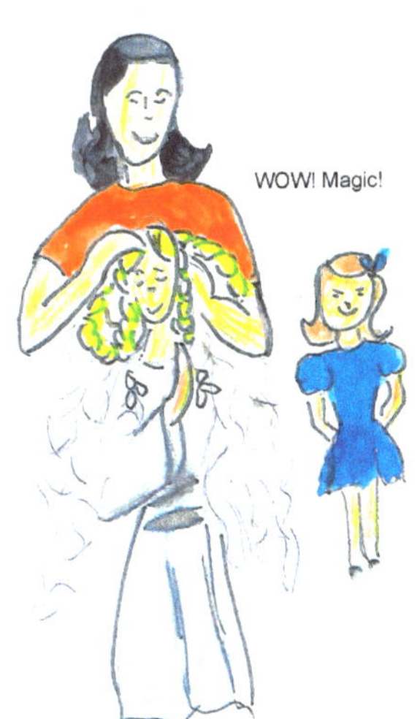

When we stopped laughing, Mom went to her chest of drawers and found a beautiful silver-gray shawl. She put my braids up like a crown around my head, pinned the shawl to my braids and arranged it around my shoulders, draped it around the old black dress, and fastened it with a lustrous pearl pin. It was wonderful. Tyke said it was magic. I ran into the bedroom to look in the mirror to see how I looked. I yelled, "WOW! Mom, you must be the good witch from *The Wizard of Oz*. Thank you, Mom. My costume is perfect."

This is the pattern

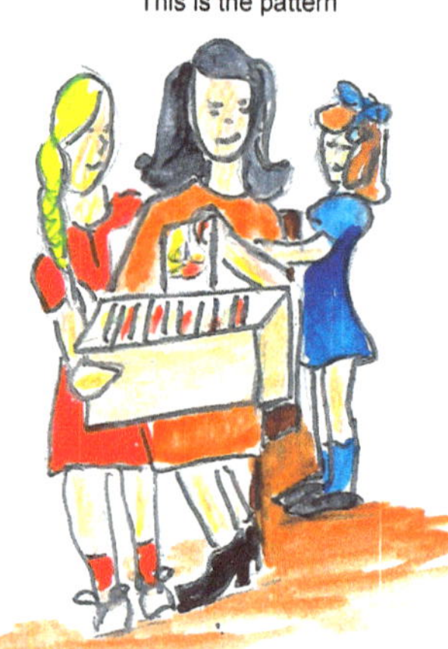

Tyke said, "Yvonne has her costume, but what nice dress am I going to wear to sing in the front row at the program?" Mom said, "I will make you a pretty new dress, and you can wear your Easter shoes." She went into the bedroom closet and brought out a sewing drawer with pink fabric and patterns for a dress Tyke's size. Tyke and I both gave Mom a big hug and another thank-you. Now we were ready for the program.

The Mother's Day program was a great success. The children practiced and were very serious about where they had to stand and how important it was to learn all the words of all the songs that they sang. The girls who played the part of the mothers had to be very serious about rocking their babies and smiling while the songs were being sung. We had a wonderful time, and the parents said they loved our program.

Mother's Day Program

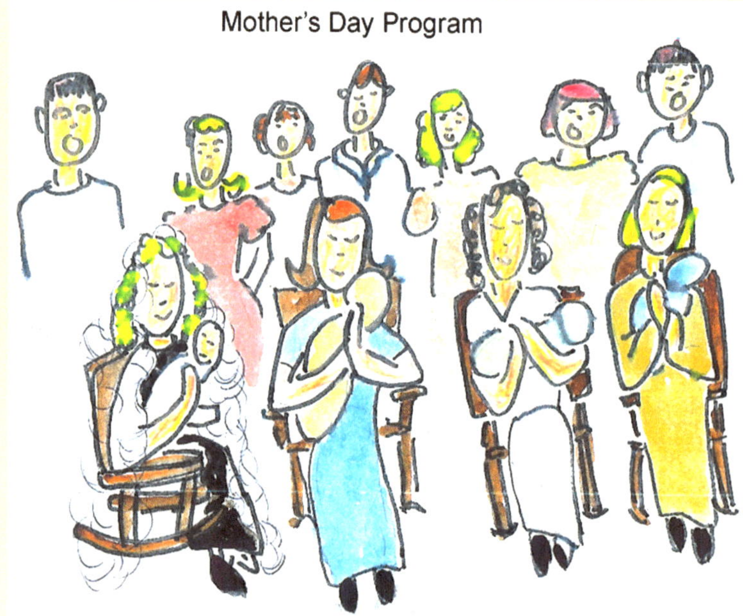

School can be great!

Chapter 21

A few weeks after the program, it was time for me to go to San Francisco. This would be my first checkup after my surgery at Stanford. My mother and I had to take the train from Portola to San Francisco to Stanford-Lane Hospital. It was a long trip. We left Portola early in the morning and arrived in Oakland late in the afternoon. When we got to Oakland, we walked to the dock and crossed the bay by ferry to San Francisco. Once we got off the ferry, we had to find a bus that would take us downtown to my father's uncle John's apartment where we would spend the night.

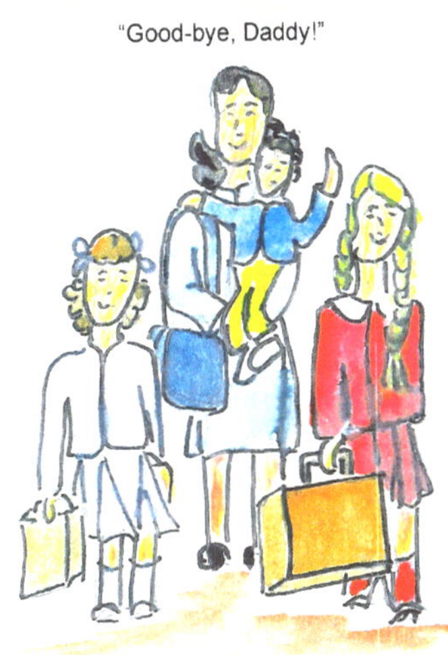

Tyke and Donnie went on the train with us as far as Sacramento. My grandmother would take my sister and brother from the train to stay at her house. Grandma would take care of them, and our cousins would visit Grandma and play with Tyke and Donnie until we come back from San Francisco. They would meet us in Sacramento, and we would all go home together.

When Mom and I got to San Francisco, we went to the apartment of my father's uncle John. Uncle John had city maps to show us what buses to take to get to the Stanford-Lane Hospital next morning. My father's uncle and aunt were very happy to see us and very kind and generous. We had dinner with them that evening. Uncle John told funny jokes to make us laugh. We had a good time, but Mom said we were tired, and so we went to bed before I was ready.

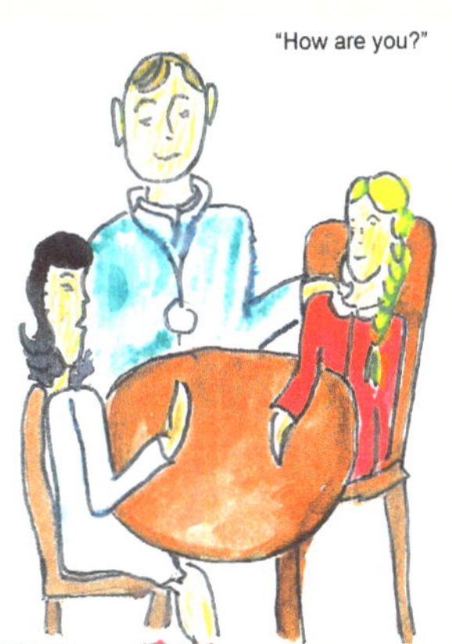

Mom and I got up early the next morning and had breakfast with Daddy's aunt and uncle. We found the right bus and went to the Stanford-Lane Hospital where we had an appointment to visit my doctor. Dr. King, the doctor in charge, did not usually come to the clinic, but he was there that day because he wanted to see how well I had done the past three months. When he saw me, he looked happy and pleased. He wanted to know how I felt—if I had been to school, if I had any friends, and what I was going to do this summer. We had a great talk. I didn't know what I was going to do this summer, but I told him about all the things that had happened. We talked about one-hour days of class to start with, when I had special reading and math classes, and where I met my new friends. I told him about falling off the rings. Some of the teachers thought it was too dangerous for me to play on the rings. We had to make new rules about handicapped kids in school. I told him that I added time to my school day by about one hour each week and was finally able to go to school all day, and I was even in the Mother's Day program at school.

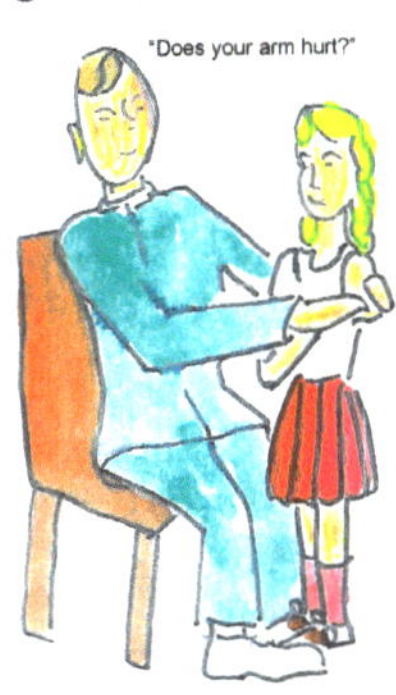

He said, "That is fantastic!" Then he said, "Let's take a look at your arm and see if it is completely healed. Does your arm hurt you?" I said, "Only if you touch where the stitches had been on the side of my arm or the bottom of the stump where you can feel the bone." "Do you have any trouble with the nerves hurting you?" I told him that sometimes I could feel my elbow and my fingers. Sometimes it really hurt. Sometimes it tingled or felt itchy. Dr. McKnight had explained to me that I should expect to feel my missing arm. He asked if I had a hard time with my balance. It had been hard at first. I bumped into the furniture and doorways. I had to be aware of objects so I could avoid bumping into everything around me. I told him I was doing pretty well now. I had hard toe ballet slippers and learned to stand on my toes and danced around the house. I could run. I told him about being a cowgirl with all my cowgirl friends on the playground at recess. I also told him I could swing on the rings and play on the monkey bars. He laughed and told me he was amazed at how well I looked and all the things I had done in the last three months. When he finished examining me, he said, "Everything has gone better than expected. Your progress is great." Then he added, "Keep up the good work. Have a great summer, and I'll see you in three months." I said, "Thank you. I will. Good-bye!"

I like cable cars!

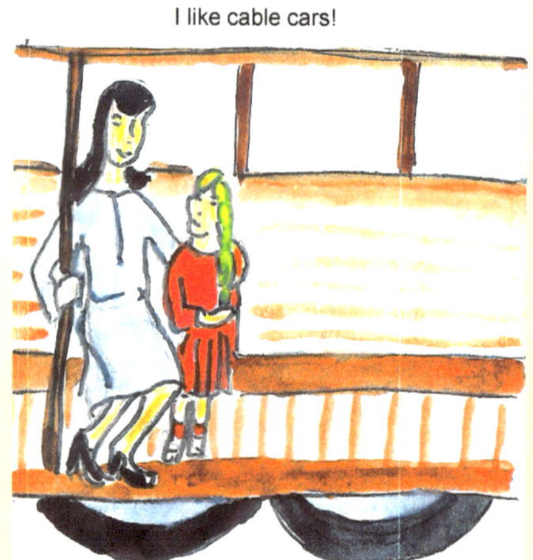

Mom and I left the hospital a little before noon. Mom asked if I was hungry, and I said yes. She said, "Let's go to Chinatown for lunch." We took the cable car to Chinatown. Just riding the cable car was worth the trip. When we got to Chinatown, we walked through all the little stores and saw many beautiful things. We bought a little china doll for Tyke and a soft toy for Donnie. Then we went to a beautifully painted building with dragons on the door—all in red and gold and green. It was a Chinese restaurant. We walked inside, and a very nice waiter bowed to us and asked us how many for lunch. Mom told him, "My daughter and I." He took us to a little chamber that had a curtain in front. He pulled back the curtain, and there was a table and two benches for us to sit on. There was a beautiful Chinese lamp hanging from the ceiling. It was painted red and gold. It had glass sides where the light shone through and little red tassels on the four corners of the lantern's frame. I thought it was magical. The waiter gave us a menu, a pot of tea, and two little cups with no handles; and then he left. Mom and I drank tea from the little cups, chose food from the menu, and soon the waiter took our order and brought our food. The food was delicious, and being with Mom in San Francisco in a cubicle in Chinatown was wonderful. When we finished lunch, Mom said, "It's time for us to begin our trip home." We stopped at Uncle John's just long enough to get our things, hugged everybody, said good-bye, and went to the ferry building.

"I love this place!"

Good-bye,
San Francisco!

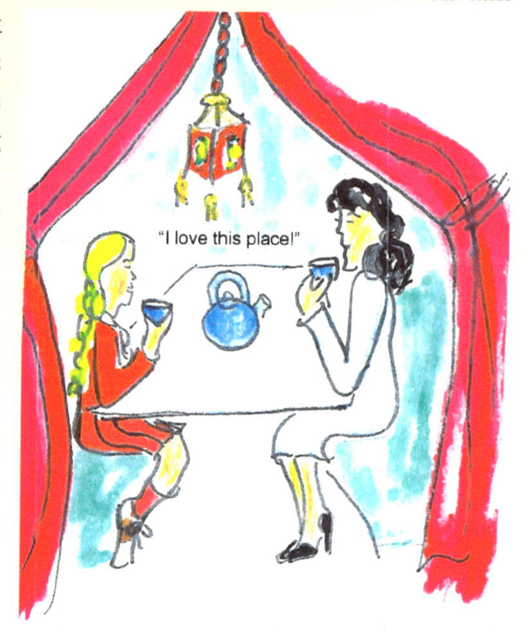

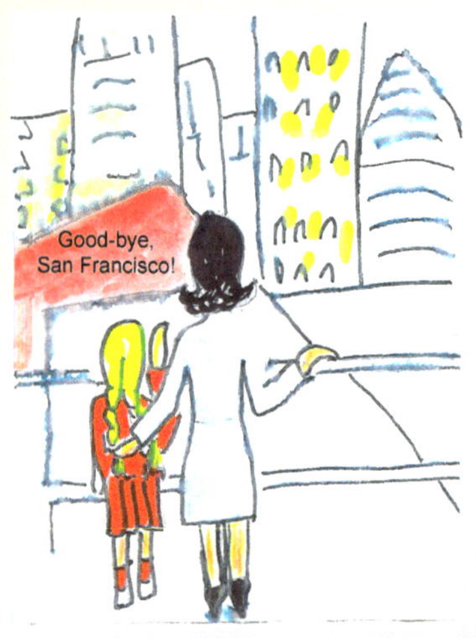

We got to the ferry building, my favorite part of the trip. I loved riding the ferry across the bay. It was fun to walk up the ramp with all the people. We walked up past different decks until we got to the top deck. We went outside on the top deck. The seagulls were all around, screeching and making lots of noise and causing excitement. The smell of the sea, the wind blowing my hair and whipping my coat around me are the things I remember as being very special. In a very short time, we were across the bay in Oakland, rushing toward the train. We got on the train, gave our tickets to the conductor, and settled down in our seats.

As the train headed for Sacramento, Mom and I sat back and relaxed. We were both more tired than we realized, and we took a little nap. We woke up just as we were leaving Stockton train station. Then we started looking for the Sacramento station where Tyke and Donnie would be waiting for us. In just a few minutes, we were pulling into the station, and there was Uncle Alfred, Grandma Souza, Tyke, and Donnie. Everybody was excited. Grandma asked how the doctor visit had gone; she wanted to know if I was all healed or if I would have to go back. Mom said that I was healed, but I would have to go to the clinic four times a year until I was grown. She explained that test cases for drugs need to be documented over a long period of time. Tyke and Donnie were talking about playing with the cousins at Grandma's house. Grandma said, "The kids were great. I loved having them. I hope you all come down and visit soon." The train whistled and slowly left the station as we waved good-bye to Grandma and Uncle Alfred.

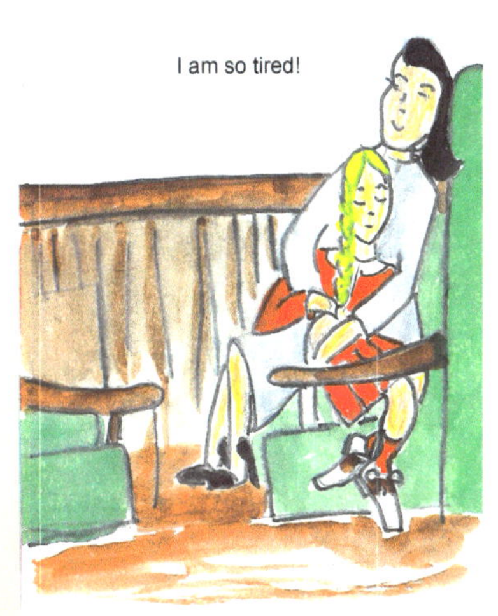

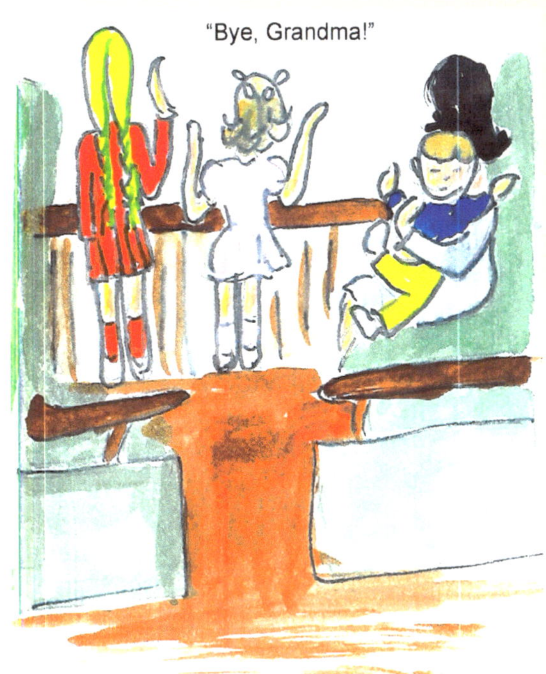

We were all glad to be together and on our way home to see Daddy.

We waved good-bye to Uncle Alfred and Grandma until we couldn't see them anymore. Then we hugged one another and listened to all the fun things Donnie and Tyke had done at Grandma's house. We told them we brought them a surprise from Chinatown. Tyke loved her doll, and Donnie played with his toy as we rode the rest of the way to Portola where Daddy would meet us.

Love is a happy, healthy family!

BIBLIOGRAPHY

Ratcliff, J. D. *Yellow Magic: The Story of Penicillin.* New York: Random House, 1945.

"Rare Penicillin Secured to Save Life of Girl," *Portola Reporter*, September 9, 1943.

"Penicillin Cures Gas Gangrene Victim," *Portola Reporter*, February 3, 1944.

"Medicine: 20th Century Seer." *Time.* May 15, 1944.

"Penicillin in Gas Gangrene: Report of a Successfully Treated Case." *The Journal of the American Medical Association* 124 (1944): 360

McKnight, W. B., Loewenberg, Richard D., and Wright, Virginia L., *The Journal of the American Association* 124 (1944): 360.

REPORT OF CASE

Y. T., a girl aged 7 years, of normal.... {Full Text PDF of this article}

Blizzard, Bill. "On Thin Ice," *Portola Reporter*, May 18, 1944.

"Elementary School Entertains Mothers with the Tea," *Portola Reporter*.

www.ingramcontent.com/pod-product-compliance
Ingram Content Group UK Ltd.
Pitfield, Milton Keynes, MK11 3LW, UK
UKHW060120300726
14090UKWH00002B/288

* 9 7 8 1 4 5 3 5 1 7 8 0 2 *